CHILD,

Towards a Knowledge Base

Second Edition

Brian Corby

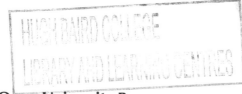
Open University Press

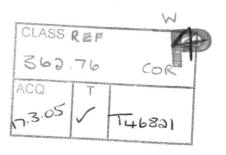

Open University Press
McGraw-Hill Education
McGraw-Hill House
Shoppenhangers Road
Maidenhead
Berkshire
SL6 2QL
United Kingdom

email: enquiries@openup.co.uk
world wide web: www.openup.co.uk

and
Two Penn Plaza
New York, NY 10121-2289, USA

First Published 1993
First published in this second edition, 2000
Reprinted 2003, 2004

A catalogue record for this book is available from the British Library.

ISBN 0 335 20568 2 (hb)   0 335 20567 4 (pb)

Library of Congress Cataloging-in-Publication Data
Corby, Brian.
    Child abuse / Brian Corby. – 2nd ed.
      p. cm.
    Includes bibliographical references and index.
    ISBN 0–335–20568–2 – ISBN 0–335–20567–4 (pbk.)
    1. Child abuse. I. Title.

HV6626.5.C67 2000
362.76–dc21   00–037507

Typeset by Graphicraft Limited, Hong Kong
Printed and bound in Great Britain by Biddles Ltd, King's Lynn, Norfolk

This book is dedicated to the memory of
Frances Mary Buchanan

CHILD **ABUSE**

Second Edition

CONTENTS

ACKNOWLEDGEMENTS

I would first of all like to thank those who were generous enough to make positive comments about the first edition of this book – this gave me the confidence to contemplate and then work on a second edition. I would next like to thank two of my colleagues at Liverpool University – Clare Minghella-Horton for all the help she gave me with various IT tasks that proved beyond my capabilities, and Malcolm Millar for pushing me to clarify certain parts of the text. Finally, I would like to thank my family again for putting up with me during the process of writing.

chapter **one**

INTRODUCTION

Since the publication of the first edition of this book in 1993, there has been a series of new developments in the field of child abuse in Britain.

There has been a considerable shift in thinking about intrafamilial child abuse and about the way in which professional intervention in such cases should be carried out. Essentially the certainty of purpose about the state's response to incidents of child abuse within the family which has previously informed many of the policy developments in this field (if not as obviously the practice of front-line professionals) is beginning to evaporate.

As was made clear in the first edition, this was starting to happen in the early 1990s following the publication of the Cleveland (Butler-Sloss 1988) and Orkney inquiry reports (Clyde 1992), both of which raised questions about the over-zealous and insensitive styles of child protection interventions into incidents of sexual and ritual abuse which featured there. This response was in sharp contrast to the findings of inquiries throughout the 1970s and most of the 1980s which had been critical of social workers' and others' responses to physical abuse and neglect cases for not being sufficiently assertive and child protectionist.

Messages from research

However, the key turning-point came in 1995 with the publication of a series of Department of Health (DoH) research projects which had been commissioned soon after the Cleveland inquiry report to examine a broad range of issues relating to child protection interventions and more general questions about the extent and consequences of child abuse and neglect.

The findings of these research initiatives were summarized in 1995 in a DoH sponsored publication *Child Protection: Messages from Research* (DoH 1995). Fuller details of the implications of this document for child protection practice will be considered in Chapter 4. The main conclusions reached were that the child protection system had become over-concerned with detecting and investigating physical and sexual abuse cases, that is the forms of abuse that were more overt or in the public eye. It was argued that in fact these forms of abuse constituted only a minority of child care concern referrals, but nevertheless dominated professionals' thinking. As a consequence of this, other referrals, especially those about families where persistently poor standards of care and neglect were prevalent, tended to be overlooked despite research showing that such 'abuse' can have the most damaging and long-lasting ill-effects of all forms of abuse.

The research summarized by *Messages from Research* also confirmed the findings of the Cleveland and Orkney inquiry reports. It drew particularly on the parents' perspectives and showed that many interventions were perceived as intrusive, stigmatic and unhelpful.

As a consequence of these findings, the *Messages from Research* document argued that there was a clear need for child protection professionals to be more discerning in their assessment of risk to children and for more attention to be paid to the quality of life provided by parents for children than to the actual abuse incidents. It also argued that a more family supportive approach was required in order to meet the needs of children living in neglectful situations of the kind described above and to engage parents more positively in the process. The more assertive child protective approach was seen to be inappropriate in most circumstances.

These developments, therefore, have created a major change in thinking about child abuse. To some degree they have raised questions about whether the child abuse label is useful in any way at all, whether child protection interventions do more harm than good and whether it might be more useful to reframe all but the very serious cases as ones requiring family support.

Children abused outside the family

Institutional abuse

While this has been the main shift in thinking about child abuse since 1993, it has not been the only one. Concerns about the abuse of children in residential care which were coming on to the agenda in the early 1990s, particularly with the publication of the Pindown report (Staffordshire 1991), have grown apace. There were ten or more major inquiries into this form of abuse throughout the 1990s and several large-scale police inquiries in different parts of the UK. Many of these are still ongoing and have resulted in the prosecution of large numbers of residential workers for cruelty and for sexual offences against the children entrusted to their care.

Paedophiles

Linked to the phenomenon of institutional abuse and also to increased knowledge about organized abuse (see Bibby 1996), the second half of the 1990s saw a massive increase in concern about paedophiles and their threat to children (usually outside the family). There has also been much more focus on younger sex offenders and latterly on the abusive aspects of child prostitution.

If one were to generalize about developments in the 1990s, one might characterize it as a period where child protection concerns shifted from intrafamilial abuse to the abuse of children outside the family, with the former gradually being reframed, except in the most serious cases, as symptoms of families failing to cope and provide adequate child care standards.

These shifts in thinking will be responded to in this second edition – indeed they are the main reason for updating the original book. The first edition focused mainly on research relating to intrafamilial physical and sexual abuse. To some degree this focus will be broadened in order to give greater consideration to current research and knowledge development about extrafamilial abuse and neglect.

Other developments

Ongoing concerns about intrafamilial child abuse

However, it is also important not to get carried away with these social and political shifts. Intrafamilial child abuse (or whatever term we use to define psychological and physical harms to children resulting from parental acts or omissions) remains an important concern for both practitioners and researchers. Since the early 1990s there has been no diminution in the quantity of research being carried out in this field, particularly in the USA. Most notably, there has been greater focus on identifying those children most at risk of being abused and also on the consequences of mistreatment for children, their future families and society as a whole. These continuing strands of research will also form part of this edition's update.

The European dimension

Finally, it should be stressed that our understanding of and responses to child abuse have in the 1990s taken more account of the wider European scene than before. There is now much more information available about the treatment of child abuse in other European countries (see Cooper *et al.* 1995; Pringle 1998) and reference to Europe will become even more important with the likelihood of greater political and social convergence in the coming years. This perspective will, therefore, be given more prominence than in the first edition.

The aims and outline of the book

To summarize, therefore, in this edition, knowledge about physical abuse, neglect and sexual abuse of children within the family will be presented again and updated where there have been significant changes. In addition, the net will be spread more widely in order to include the newer concerns and emphases outlined above.

Philosophically, the intention of the second edition remains the same as that of the first, to concentrate primarily on providing a critically informed knowledge base for child protection workers. It is worth reiterating that this is not a how-to-do-it book. The focus remains on a broad range of sources of knowledge about the mistreatment of children, drawing on research and theorizing carried out in a variety of professional and academic disciplines: social work, medicine, history, sociology, philosophy, social policy and psychology. Increasingly child protection policy and practice seem to be centrally defined by a string of government publications. If this perception is an accurate one, then it seems even more important to bring together knowledge about child abuse from a broader base.

In most other ways, the aims of the original book remain, that is to present up-to-date research-based knowledge in a critical way, evaluating its strengths and weaknesses, and giving particular attention to how the values and beliefs of researchers influence their findings. I remain committed to a model of the social worker (and other child protection professionals) developing specialist expertise in child abuse work, and having a fair degree of autonomy in their practice. There is a distinct possibility that in the light of developments outlined above there may be increasing opportunities for this to happen as practitioners are required to be more flexible and discerning in their assessments and provision of family support. A counter-trend to this is the increased involvement of central government referred to above and the resultant effect of top-down management of these new developments.

The overall format of the book remains the same as that of the first edition. In Chapter 2 the focus is on how, throughout history, there have been different constructions and understandings of what constitutes childhood and child abuse. It is argued that careful analysis of historical research can help in the understanding of the present.

Chapters 3 and 4 concentrate on the recent history of child protection policy and practice up to the present time. Detailed consideration is given to how social and political forces have shaped the way in which we respond to child abuse allegations today. The aim is to help those currently involved in this field of activity to understand the reasons for the complex and often contradictory nature of that response.

Chapter 5 considers the issue of child abuse definition, and the impact of different definitions on policy, practice and research.

Chapter 6 looks at research into the incidence and prevalence of child abuse. It is argued that by developing a sense of the whole, practitioners can acquire a more realistic view of their particular roles and functions.

Chapter 7 looks critically at research into the question of who is likely to abuse whom and in what circumstances. Knowledge of this research is seen to be of crucial importance for those trying to assess and make decisions about cases of child abuse.

Chapter 8 considers a range of social and psychological theories and ideologies that have been applied to child abuse to explain why it happens. It is argued that understanding why abuse may be happening is an important precursor to planning intervention to prevent its recurrence.

Chapter 9 reviews research into the consequences and aftermath of abuse of children. This research has implications for both the practice and the policy of ongoing child protection work, which at present is heavily focused on the detection and investigation stages.

Chapter 10 describes empirical research into child protection practice, including in particular Department of Health research published in 1995 and 1996. The impact of research on policy and practice is particularly emphasized.

Chapter 11 considers some of the major issues that currently beset workers and researchers in the child protection field.

chapter **two**

CHILDHOOD, CHILD ABUSE AND HISTORY

Social work is a very present-oriented activity. The social work profession is committed to tackling current social and personal problems and is concerned to find useful and pragmatic tools to help in this endeavour. Indeed, in its determination to discover solutions it has been criticized for being too ready to adopt fashionable new theories and approaches (Howe 1980). This here-and-now emphasis has contributed to a lack of enthusiasm for a historical understanding of social problems and responses to them. This lack of enthusiasm is illustrated by the fact that there are few good historical accounts of the profession itself.[1]

If we consider the specific field of child protection work, this ignorance of the past is all too evident. Most social work accounts of the background to child protection work begin with Henry Kempe and his 'discovery' of the child battering syndrome in the early 1960s (Kempe *et al.* 1962), as if the problem either did not exist before this or had somehow lain dormant. Similarly, sexual abuse is often described as having been discovered in Britain at the beginning of the 1980s. However, to take just one example, accounts of the child protection movement in the late nineteenth and early twentieth centuries, such as those by Behlmer (1982), Rose (1986, 1991) and Ferguson (1990), demonstrate that very similar things were happening in this field then as are happening today, albeit in a very different social context and climate. Infant life protection protagonists, National Society for the Prevention of Cruelty to Children (NSPCC) officials and various other philanthropic agents were then emphasizing the widespread nature of child abuse and seeking to convince the public of the need for a change in attitude. In the same way as social workers today, they were decrying the fact that the law was woefully deficient in dealing with the problem and arguing vehemently that children should be more adequately protected. The experiences of these late Victorians, considered in more detail in Chapter 3, in fact provide us with a rich source of useful material for evaluating contemporary responses to child protection issues. As we shall see, however, in order to benefit from this type of approach we have to interpret the historian's word as critically and as objectively as possible.

Interpreting history

Historians themselves are well aware of the difficulties of learning from the past:

> The study of past attitudes, of modes of thought and feeling is one of the most difficult branches of historiography. Not only is evidence patchy and often indirect, particularly where intimate family matters or the mentality of the inarticulate or the illiterate

are concerned, but the interpretation of such evidence requires an empathy, a feeling for nuances, and above all an objectivity, a deliberate attempt to set aside one's own cultural assumptions that is not easy to attain . . . Huge generalisations have been hoisted on the slenderest foundations, evidence that is not congenial has been ignored or brushed aside, while other testimony has been crudely or carelessly misinterpreted. All of which suggests the need for a reminder that bad history can still mislead the 'general public' as well as other scholars and students.

(Wilson 1984: 198)

All historical writing is inevitably selective. The range of sources available is often vast. Historians have their favoured viewpoints and theories, which influence the way in which they interpret data, and this results in emphasis on certain types of evidence and lack of attention to others. For instance, historical writing varies considerably with regard to the attention paid to the different forms of structural oppression, such as race, class, gender and age and their impact on attitudes and behaviours. Currently there is considerable reassessment of the past through these filters, particularly in the case of race and gender.

When history is used as a means of casting light on present issues, there seem to be two mainstream perspectives. The first views the present as an inevitable improvement on the past. Adherents of this viewpoint draw comfort from the ignorance and mistakes (as they see them) of previous generations. The second paints a rosy picture of yesteryear and sees the present not as progress from the past, but as retrogressive. The first perspective views the past as barbaric, the second as a golden age. It is important to be aware of and to understand different viewpoints of this kind in order to maximize the usefulness of historical material.

Childhood and history

The issues of childhood and child abuse are closely linked. Views about the status and rights of children have considerable influence on the way in which they are treated by adults and determine to some extent what is considered to be mistreatment. For the purposes of analysis, however, they will be treated separately. This section will consider what historians tell us about childhood.

Childhood as a social construct

While it may not solve the immediate question of whether social workers should apply for an emergency protection order in the case of a young child left alone and unprotected, or whether they should try to rehabilitate a teenage child who is rejecting his or her parents, awareness of the socially constructed nature of childhood can enable social workers to reflect more fully on the social and political under-pinnings to the situation and may ultimately inform the decisions that are finally reached in these and other cases. As one historian puts it:

> One possible spin-off of a historical approach is that it can pre-vent us from taking any particular set of attitudes or behaviours as 'natural' or 'normal'. By examining the historical variety of the position of children and of ideas about childhood and by tracing back some of the steps by which we arrived at our present situ-ation, we can achieve a more dispassionate analysis.
>
> (Jordanova 1989: 4–5)

To the lay person the notion of childhood is self-evident. Everyone knows a child when they see one. Of course it becomes a little more difficult in the case of adolescents. Nevertheless, most people consider childhood to be an age-related phenomenon. This is reflected in Brit-ish law, which prescribes a series of legal rights and responsibilities that take effect at different ages. These statutes provide protection for children, place duties on their parents, impose prohibitions on certain activities and later lift them. There are all sorts of anomalies. For instance, in the UK a 16-year-old is deemed responsible enough to marry (with parental consent) and have children, but not responsible enough to buy an alcoholic drink in a public house or to watch a category 18 film. Heterosexuals can consent to sexual acts at the age of 16, but homosexual males cannot do so until they are aged 18 (reduced from 21 in 1994). A boy can legally consent to sexual inter-course at 14, but girls cannot do so until they are 16. While the age of 18 is generally thought to be the beginning of adulthood, there are still prohibitions which last until the age of 21. Only then can a young person stand as a councillor or Member of Parliament (MP), apply for a licence to sell alcohol, have a heavy goods vehicle licence or apply to adopt a child. Such is the power of chronological age.

Despite these tightly age-related demarcations, we know that chil-dren develop and mature, both physically and psychologically, at dif-ferent rates. We also know that in societies other than our own childhood is construed differently. In many countries in the southern hemisphere, childhood is mostly shorter, particularly if a child is poor, black and female (see Ennew 1986). Children generally assume what we would term adult responsibilities at an earlier age in these societies than in northern industrially developed countries, where childhood has tended to be extended to higher and higher ages. The trend in these northern countries is to keep young people in education longer, because of the reduced demand for manual labour and the increased demand for a better trained workforce as technology and markets develop and become more complex.

Historians seem to have paid far more attention to children and the concept of childhood since the 1960s than ever before. This may well reflect the apparent growth in concerns about children and childhood in contemporary society during this period. Even here, however, we need to be careful in our interpretations. Sommerville (1982) demonstrates that in Mesopotamia in 1800 BC parents were expressing the same sort of concerns about their children as parents are now, that is that they were not obedient and that they were not working hard enough at school. Concerns about children, therefore, seem to be perennial ones. Nevertheless, it is true that since the 1960s we do have a great deal more historical material to draw upon than before.

Philippe Ariès and childhood

The most influential work on childhood of this period has been that of Philippe Ariès, a French social historian. He, along with Lloyd De Mause, an American psychohistorian, whose work is considered later (see pp. 13–16), is probably the most often quoted historian in child care textbooks. The popular view put forward by social work writers of Ariès's ideas (with one notable exception – Frost and Stein 1989) is that the notion of childhood is a relatively recent one (a product of the seventeenth century). This is usually used to show that we have become more sensitive to children and their needs than was true in the past. Strangely this is almost a total misreading of what Ariès was arguing. In *Centuries of Childhood,* Ariès (1962) wrote:

> In medieval society the idea of childhood did not exist: this is not to suggest that children were neglected, forsaken or despised. The idea of childhood is not to be confused with affection for children: it corresponds to an awareness of the particular nature of childhood, that particular nature which distinguishes the child from the adult, even the young adult. In medieval society this awareness was lacking.
>
> (Ariès 1962: 125)

Ariès did not see the absence of the concept of childhood as detrimental to children. Indeed he thought the opposite to be true. During the Middle Ages, according to him, children mingled with adults as soon as that was physically possible. They spent much of their time together in both work and play. It was only gradually, and most dramatically in the seventeenth century with the advent of a form of education dominated by religion-based morality, that children became separated from adults in the way that we understand it today. This increasing differentiation of children from adults in the public sphere was seen by Ariès as a backward step, that is it served to place greater restrictions on children in their formative years. The concept of childhood is not seen by him as improving children's status, but as a limiting force placing children more at the mercy of adults than had previously been the case. Ariès can be seen, therefore, as a child liberationist. He would like to undo the chains imposed by this modern concept of childhood and return to a more varied, open and liberated past.

Many historians, however, do not find Ariès's account of the development of childhood to be plausible (see Hunt 1970; Hanawalt 1977; Hoyles 1979; Macfarlane 1979; Thane 1981; Pollock 1983; Wilson 1984; Boswell 1990). Pollock (1983) summarizes the criticisms of his work in her excellent study, *Forgotten Children*. Her main argument is that Ariès's sources of evidence are not sufficient to back his wide-ranging claims. First, he placed heavy reliance on paintings that could have been analysed in a variety of ways, although he interpreted them only in ways that supported his views. His second main source was Heroard's diary of the early years of the future Louis XIII of France. He used this work, which shows Louis to have been regarded and reared as a little man from a very early age, particularly in terms of sexuality, to demonstrate his general thesis of the non-existence of childhood at that time. Pollock's (1983) view is that this case is atypical and tells us very little about how children in general were viewed and treated at this time. This seems to be a reasonable criticism: consider to what extent the diary of Prince Charles's nanny (assuming that she wrote one) would give people in the twenty-fourth century a true flavour of European child-rearing practices in the twentieth century.

Pollock (1983) is critical of Ariès's rather rosy view of family life in the Middle Ages, which suggests full integration of children and adults into an idealized communal life. She also points out that Ariès has nothing to say about the care of children who are still physically dependent on their parents. He gives the impression that until children are aged 7 they do not count (it is almost as if they have no existence at all) and that once they reach this age they are fully mature and are assimilated into adult life without any problems.

The disputes over Ariès's work highlight the potential benefits and dangers of a historical perspective on children's issues. He clearly sensitizes us to the fact that childhood is a social construction and that the 'problems' of childhood can be socially created. However, he is deficient in terms of explaining why this happens and makes rather sweeping statements on the basis of limited sources. As Wilson (1984: 183) points out: 'Unfortunately, Ariès expressed himself more categorically than he might have done, and he attracted followers, rather than critics, initially.'

The barbaric past perspective

Many historians have used Ariès's argument that childhood did not exist until the seventeenth century to show that in fact children have been subject to, at the least, detached emotional upbringings and, at the most, severe abuse including infanticide (see Plumb 1975; De Mause 1976; Shorter 1976; Stone 1977; Badinter 1981). De Mause in particular makes this claim. His argument is that the more remote the period of history being examined, the more cruel the treatment of children becomes.

> The history of childhood is a nightmare from which we have only recently begun to awaken. The further back in history one goes, the lower the level of child care, and the more likely children are to be killed, abandoned, beaten, terrorised and sexually abused.
>
> (De Mause 1976: 1)

De Mause therefore shares with Ariès the belief that childhood is a product of relatively recent times, but there the similarity of view ends. Whereas Ariès sees the development of the concept of childhood as repressive, De Mause sees it as highly progressive. For him childhood has evolved from the dark ages to the golden present. He outlines seven evolutionary stages ranging from what he terms the infanticidal mode, which existed until the fourth century, to the helping mode, which commenced in the middle of the twentieth century. Gradually over generations of evolution, we have progressed, according to De Mause, from a state where parents were unable to see their children as separate beings with any particular needs, to that where they regard them as distinct, different and deserving of a special set of rights that emphasize respect for them as full human beings.

Stone (1977), focusing on the 1500–1800 period, provides some support for this type of thesis. He argues that affection and love between spouses and for their children were impossible before the eighteenth century because of the material conditions of pre-industrial life. Adults did not invest emotionally in children because it was not considered to be worthwhile. Child mortality rates were so high that 'to preserve their mental stability, parents were obliged to limit the degree of their psychological involvement with their infant children' (Stone 1977: 70). It was only in the nineteenth century, in his view, that children were first seen as individuals with special needs because of their vulnerability. This change in perception stemmed initially from the upper and middle classes, who had acquired more leisure time to devote to child care concerns, and was gradually filtered down to the poorer classes.

These and similar views have been heavily criticized by other historians. Demos (1986) is critical of De Mause for the selectivity of his material and the fact that he seems to totally ignore the context and, therefore, the meaning of the behaviours which he is condemning. Macfarlane's (1979) review of Stone's work is particularly telling. He quotes many examples of parents expressing love and affection for their children before the eighteenth century. In particular Macfarlane (1970) refers to the diary of a seventeenth-century Puritan vicar, Ralph Josselin, and the grief that he expresses at the death of his 8-year-old daughter, Mary.[2] Macfarlane (1979) argues that Stone (1977) ignores evidence from modern societies in the southern hemisphere and from social anthropological studies that demonstrate considerable evidence of close child–adult emotional ties despite gross material poverty and high rates of child mortality. Macfarlane does not accept Stone's neat evolutionary scheme and is unconvinced by his belief that affective relationships are determined totally by economics.

There is a growing body of evidence to suggest that the concept of childhood as a status eliciting a form of response and treatment different to that of adults has always existed. Boswell (1990: 37) in his study of abandonment of children in antiquity argues: 'It is clear, however, that there was no general absence of tender feeling for children as special beings among any premodern European peoples.' Houlbrooke (1984), writing about families in the fifteenth century, states:

> Children were seen by many as an important source of help and comfort in old age. To all save those engaged in the most brutal struggle for mere survival, they were probably a source of psychological satisfaction which varied in depth according to the individual character.
>
> (Houlbrooke 1984: 127)

Somewhat more cynically, he says that 'parents delighted in their children, not primarily because of their good qualities, but because they were theirs' (Houlbrooke 1984: 135).

Pollock (1983), drawing from a study of 496 published diaries and autobiographies written between 1500 and 1900, argues that the concept of childhood changed and developed during this period but certainly existed throughout. The sources which she considered all demonstrated a certain amount of ambivalence towards their children. All saw them as a mixture of good and bad or of innocence and depravity. All demonstrated human concern and a sense of responsibility, as well as finding their children wearisome and exasperating. In particular, the diaries she examined showed that the death of a child created the same heartfelt reactions throughout the centuries studied.

It must be concluded, therefore, that although there is no doubt that children in former times were expected to work and become what we today would consider to be adult at an earlier age than our own children, claims regarding the non-existence of the notion of childhood as we perceive it now are grossly exaggerated. It seems likely that children have always had a separate status, particularly early on when they are more physically dependent. As societies develop economically there is a tendency for childhood to be extended and to gain more attention as a separate category, a process that is testified to by the growth of child protective legislation.

A major flaw in many historical analyses of childhood is that they tend to generalize about the way in which children are perceived (and, therefore, behave and are treated), as if all children's experiences are similar at a particular time. It is highly likely that this is far from true. Children of different classes, genders and races are likely to have widely different experiences in every period of history. A good example of this variation in experience is provided by the period of industrialization in Britain in the nineteenth century, during which the development of greater sensitivity and sentiment towards middle-class childhood coincided with appalling working conditions for children of the labouring classes in mills, factories and on the street (see Davin 1990).

Child abuse and history

What do historians tell us about child abuse? The existence of child mistreatment in history (infanticide, abandonment, severe physical chastisement, child prostitution and harsh labour) is indisputable. The extent of such mistreatment and the interpretation of it within the societies where it took place are issues of greater contention. As we shall see, some historians consider that the vast majority of children in the past were callously treated and that this was seen as relatively normal because there was little sense of childhood as a protected status. Other historians take the view that extreme ill-treatment of children was not as common in recorded history as argued by the above, and that while general standards of care for children were lower than what we expect today, largely because of harsh economic conditions, gross maltreatment was never accepted as normal. From this point of view it is argued that within the prevailing standards of each age there have been cruel and loving parents and that children who had cruel parents were likely to be abused, but society did not necessarily condone or accept such abuse.

Cruel treatment of children in antiquity

De Mause (1976) placed the Roman empire in his infanticide mode. Infanticide was not legally a crime until AD 318 (made punishable by death in AD 374). De Mause concludes from this that it was not only common practice but also evidence of the cruelty of the times. Boswell, whose study *The Kindness of Strangers* (1990) is concerned with abandonment rather than infanticide, a distinction he is keen to maintain, is far less critical of the mores of this period. Whereas De Mause (1976) judges the Romans by the standards of the late twentieth century (using psychoanalytic theory as his baseline), Boswell (1990) takes into account the meaning of forms of behaviour that on the face of it seem barbaric but are more understandable under closer scrutiny. That the Romans practised infanticide is without doubt. However, seen in the light of the fact that there were no adequate contraceptive techniques and the medical knowledge needed for abortion did not exist, it becomes clear that much (not all) infanticide was a crude, though not altogether callous, means of controlling family size. Another method of achieving this was the abandonment of children. Boswell (1990) demonstrates that abandonment was many times more popular than infanticide for two reasons. First, the average Roman probably took no more pleasure in killing new-born babies than you or I would. Second, abandonment, which was usually carried out in a public place, frequently led to a child being rescued and looked after by someone else. This was in most cases a desired and intended outcome.[3]

Boswell's (1990) sympathetic account of the process of abandonment contrasts sharply with the more lurid views of De Mause (1976).

> Parents abandoned their offspring in desperation when they were unable to support them, due to poverty or disaster; in shame when they were unwilling to keep them because of their physical condition or ancestry (e.g. illegitimate or incestuous); in self-interest or the interest of another child, when inheritance or domestic resources would be compromised by another mouth; in hope, when they believed that someone of greater means or higher standing might find them and bring them up in better circumstances; in resignation, when a child was of unwelcome gender or ominous auspices; or in callousness, if they simply could not be bothered with parenthood.
>
> (Boswell 1990: 428)

Child cruelty in the Middle Ages

Boswell's study goes through to the Renaissance period. He argues that throughout Europe abandonment continued to be a common practice, never openly approved of, but never officially outlawed. Gradually the Church became more involved and began to organize and regulate the activity. Monasteries provided havens for unwanted children through the practice of oblation. In the early thirteenth century, foundling homes were established and the process of abandonment became centralized on these institutions. However, what are seen as progressive developments do not always achieve their intended goals. Boswell (1990) argued that the death rate through disease in these places was probably higher than that resulting from the previous practice of abandonment.

How common infanticide was during this period is uncertain. Although it was prohibited by ecclesiastical law in most European societies at this time, there is much evidence to show that it was a not uncommon occurrence. Shahar (1990) comments:

> The scope of the phenomenon cannot be gauged, but the number of cases was certainly too great for all of them to be attributed to murderous impulses resulting from *post partum* depression or other grave mental disturbances (although these factors were certainly involved in some cases).
>
> (Shahar 1990: 127)

Shahar also notes that the murder of children other than new-borns was very rare. Sharpe (1984) points out that by the sixteenth century infanticide was singled out for severe punishment by most European states and comments that 'The infanticide wave in England at least may have resulted in more executions than the more familiar witch craze' (Sharpe 1984: 61). The state's concern for child welfare also encompassed accidents in the home. Hanawalt (1977) refers to synodal legislation of the thirteenth century that tells parents not to sleep with their children and not to leave them alone or unattended near fires.

Sexual abuse of children in antiquity and the Middle Ages

There is little clear evidence about sexual abuse of children in antiquity and medieval times. Again De Mause is unequivocal about the former: 'The child in antiquity lived his earliest years in an atmosphere of sexual abuse. Growing up in Greece or Rome often included being sexually used by older men' (De Mause 1976: 43). Wiedemann (1989) is equally unequivocal in holding a contrary position:

> Nor for that matter do the occasional references to the sexual exploitation of children by perverts prove that Roman society as a whole was imbued either with a psychotic hatred of childhood, or with a degree of sexual freedom to put modern California to shame.
>
> (Wiedemann 1989: 30)

He points out that pederasty was not acceptable to the Romans and that if it involved a boy of citizen status it was apparently a criminal offence.[4]

Turning to intrafamilial abuse, it is clear that the Greeks and Romans operated a strict incest taboo. Sophocles' *Oedipus Rex* displays the horrors that accompanied unwitting incest. Boswell's (1990) study of abandonment was inspired by an inscription he read which warned men that by going to brothels they might be committing incest with children whom they had abandoned years before. Such fears and anxieties demonstrate how deep-seated the taboo really was.

However, we simply do not know to what extent sexual abuse of children either within or outside families was a feature in ancient societies. This is hardly surprising. As we shall see in Chapter 6, it was only in the 1980s and 1990s that there has been a concerted attempt to focus on intrafamilial sexual abuse in Britain and the USA and to try to measure its true extent.

Unsurprisingly, therefore, there is also very little information on the subject of sexual abuse during the Middle Ages period. Incest did not become a legal offence in England until the twentieth century (except for a brief period during the regency of Cromwell). However, it should not be assumed that the absence of legislation meant a lack of concern about or acceptance of such behaviour. Prior to this more secular century, the Church played a lead role in policing sexuality in England for nearly two millennia through the pulpit, the confessional and ultimately the ecclesiastical courts (see Gagnon and Parker 1995). By contrast incest was a crime punishable by death in Scotland from 1757. However policed, it is clear that the incest taboo persisted throughout Europe in this period.

Child abuse from the Middle Ages to Victorian times

Evidence for this period is as scanty as that for earlier ages. Demos (1986) carried out a study of court records in New England in the seventeenth century and found a conspicuous absence of child abuse cases. Such a finding is usually attributed to the belief that cruelty to children in this period of history was so much the norm that court action was a rarity. Demos argues that this could not have been the case because he also found several instances of master–servant violence, which resulted in action being taken to prevent its continuation. He comes to the conclusion that child abuse was probably less prevalent in New England village communities at this time than it is generally in the USA today. He attributes this to the fact that then there were larger and less introverted and intense families, children's labour value was high, filial duty was greater and there was more communal oversight of families.[5] This study runs counter to the generally held belief, put forward by De Mause (1976) and others, that child abuse inevitably declines with social progress.

Pollock (1983) demonstrated that public concern about cruelty to children in Britain existed well before the time it is generally thought to have been discovered, that is in the last three decades of the nineteenth century. She carried out a study of child cruelty reports in *The Times* between 1785 and 1860 and found 385 tried cases of child neglect, physical and sexual abuse, of which only 27 (7 per cent) were found not guilty. She commented:

> The manner in which the cases were reported by the newspaper provides an indication of the attitudes of the time to cruelty to children. The fact that the majority of the cases were also found guilty meant that law and society condemned child abuse long before the specific Prevention of Cruelty to Children Act in 1889. Parents who abused their offspring were generally considered 'unnatural' and the cruelty as 'horrific' or 'barbaric'.
>
> (Pollock 1983: 93)

However, there can be little doubt that the lot of the large numbers of children of the very poor in the seventeenth, eighteenth and early nineteenth centuries was a cruel one by present-day standards even though the cruelty was not inflicted by the parents. The accounts of the opening of the London Foundling Hospital in 1741 (McClure 1981) and of the conditions for children in workhouses at the end of the eighteenth century (Cunningham 1991) are just two reminders of the harsh reality of life for these generations of deprived children.

Concluding comments

This brief excursion into the early history of child abuse can of course prove nothing definitely. However, it should dispel at least two commonly held beliefs: first, the notion that the further one goes back in history the worse the treatment of children; second, that it is only in recent times that societies such as ours have taken concerted steps to deal with the problem.

With regard to the first point, there is no doubt that there was much harsh treatment of children in previous eras that would not be tolerated now. Nor is there any doubt that present-day children as a whole are more likely to survive infancy and enjoy better health than their predecessors as a result of medical, hygienic and material advances. On the other hand, there is evidence that children in every era have been valued, cared for, nurtured and not ill-treated. There can be no doubt that, as was stressed at the start of this chapter, many historians and social work writers have underestimated the degree of concern that parents of previous generations have shown for their children. More discerning analyses of the treatment of children in the past, such as that of Demos (1986), point to the conclusion that there are no guarantees that the quality of all children's lives will automatically improve with time.

On the second point, there is ample evidence of official concern and state action to protect children from abuse by the parents provided by historians such as Boswell (1990), Hanawalt (1977) and Demos (1986). However, this evidence seems to go unnoticed. This blindness to the efforts of previous generations to regulate cruelty to children by their parents is perhaps explained by the fact that each new generation needs to think that it is improving on the past.

Careful analysis of the history of child abuse can serve to dispel myths and to put current problems into perspective. What emerges is that every society has to deal with the issue of the care of its young and has devised some means of intervention into family life to ensure this. These efforts have been influenced by the cultures, material circumstances, technologies and politics impinging on those societies. Examining these efforts with due regard to these contextual factors can enhance our understanding of current approaches to the problem.

Recommended reading

Ariès, P. (1962) *Centuries of Childhood*. Harmondsworth: Penguin.
Boswell, J. (1990) *The Kindness of Strangers: The Abandonment of Children in Western Europe from Late Antiquity to the Renaissance*. New York: Vintage.
Cunningham, H. (1991) *Children of the Poor*. Oxford: Blackwell.
De Mause, L. (ed.) (1976) *The History of Childhood*. London: Souvenir Press.
Pollock, L. (1983) *Forgotten Children: Parent–Child Relations from 1500 to 1900*. Cambridge: Cambridge University Press.
Shahar, S. (1990) *Childhood in the Middle Ages*. London: Routledge.
Wiedemann, T. (1989) *Adults and Children in the Roman Empire*. London: Routledge.

chapter **three**

A HISTORY OF CHILD ABUSE
AND NEGLECT 1870–1991

As we saw in Chapter 2, child abuse is not a new phenomenon, nor is public or state concern about it. Nevertheless, fresh attempts to tackle child mistreatment are usually accompanied by the declaration that it is a new and as yet undiscovered problem. This 'newness' is seen as an important part of the process of establishing it as an issue requiring resources to tackle it. Often what is new about the problem is the way in which it is being defined or interpreted. This in turn can be linked to wider issues and concerns in society. In this chapter, the focus will be on responses to child abuse between 1870 and 1991, with particular attention being paid to the way in which social, economic and political forces have shaped these responses. This starting date is chosen because there is a clear thread of social organization around the problem of child abuse between then and now, and not because there was no problem or societal response to it before that.

Late Victorian and Edwardian responses to child abuse

The late Victorian age saw a flurry of activity around the issue of child protection of a similar degree and nature to that which has taken place in modern times since the early 1970s.

Socio-economic factors

Throughout the nineteenth century there were dramatic changes in terms of population growth, industrialization and urbanization in Britain. Between 1801 and 1861 the population doubled to a total of 20 million, of whom 7 million were under the age of 15. By 1901 the population was 32.5 million, of whom 10.5 million were under the age of 15. Children formed one-third of the population throughout most of this period compared with one-fifth at the present time. Even so, infant mortality rates were around 15 per cent throughout most of the nineteenth century. Rose (1991: 2) tells us: 'Even as late as 1895 half the children up to 5 would die in the worst slums, compared with 19% in a healthy district like Dulwich.'

Until the passing of the 1880 Education Act, when schooling became compulsory for children up to the age of 10, the children of the poor were likely to spend more time labouring than being educated. The 1861 census showed that one-third of all children aged 5 to 9 and nearly 50 per cent of 10- to 14-year-olds were working. Figures for working-class children alone, had they been collated, would have been much higher.

By any measure, the nineteenth century was a time of great upheaval and traumatic change for poor families and their children. These demographic changes, created largely by the demands of new technologies, led to new problems and concerns about the upbringing of children and new forms of state intervention into family life.

Child care concerns up to 1870

There had been four categories of children causing concern to the state up to the end of the 1860s: children of the street (vagabonds, beggars, street traders), young offenders, children at work and children looked after by the Poor Law authorities. The main pattern of response had been for issues to be initially taken up by philanthropic societies of different religious persuasions acting as pressure groups, followed by government intervention and state legislation (see Dingwall *et al.* 1984).

None of these child care issues involved direct intervention in the internal workings of the family. Although there was considerable concern to control the unruliness of children on the street (prompted by public order anxieties) and to influence the nature and amount of work that children were expected to undertake (prompted by concerns about exposure to immorality as well as by concerns about exploitation), there was little thought given at this time to more direct state intervention into family life to protect children from illtreatment by their parents, other than the sort of court action described by Pollock (1983), and mentioned in Chapter 2. Behlmer's (1982: 9) analysis of the situation then was that 'To patrol industry on behalf of the young was England's Christian duty. To patrol the home was a sacrilege.' While this analysis is generally correct, it is important to note that the sacrosanctity of domestic privacy to which Behlmer refers had always been more applicable to wealthier families than to those of the poor. In the pre-industrialized period the latter were subject to Church and community controls. The breakdown in these mechanisms that accompanied industrialization created a need for new ways of maintaining moral and social order among poor families, which is where the philanthropists came in. The issue for them and for the state was how best to establish this new form of intervention without undermining parents' responsibility for their children.

Baby farming

In the late 1860s and early 1870s this new form of state intervention into family affairs began tentatively, with its focus on the issue of baby farming. This term was used to describe the then common practice of paying for babies to be nursed and reared by substitute parents – the forerunner of today's private foster parents. The practice was widespread because of the absence of adequate contraceptive devices, the illegality of abortion, the stigma attached to illegitimacy and the need for poorer unmarried women to be free to work. The trade was created by unwanted pregnancies. It was a free-market enterprise uncontrolled by state surveillance. While many of the women who undertook this work may have been honest and trustworthy, there were several infamous cases of babies being murdered by their 'carers', which created widespread public concern (see Rose 1986).

The medical profession played a leading role in this issue. In 1870 the Infant Life Protection Society was established with a view to controlling the practice of baby farming by means of a system of registration and inspection. By 1872, this pressure group had succeeded in pushing through the Infant Life Protection Act, which required any adult who 'fostered' more than one child under the age of 1 year to register with the local authority and to meet certain required standards. In practice this Act proved ineffective as the resources needed to police it were not made available. London County Council was the only authority to take it at all seriously, and it appointed one inspector in 1878 to cover the whole of the metropolitan area! Further Acts dealing with this issue followed: the 1897 Infant Life Protection Act, the 1908 Children Act and the 1933 Children and Young Persons Act. The main developments were that registration was required for the first child placed, the protected age was raised to 9 and inspection, largely by health visitors, was made more thorough and comprehensive.

The Infant Life Protection Society's concern with baby farming, though seen by some as unnecessary state interference into domestic arrangements, did not meet massive resistance from the establishment. The reason for this is that it was seen as an issue that was only marginal to family life.

The formation of the NSPCC

It was not to be long before the so-called bastions of the family were to be more directly assaulted. The 1880s saw the emergence of the

Liverpool Society for the Prevention of Cruelty to Children (SPCC) and then the London SPCC (later to form the core of the National Society for the Prevention of Cruelty to Children). Most of the larger conurbations in Britain followed suit soon after. While other philanthropic societies, such as Dr Barnardo's, had been 'rescuing' children living outside their families, the SPCC's concern was to 'rescue' children living in their own homes.

The early SPCC protagonists considered existing arrangements for the reporting of child ill-treatment and neglect and the subsequent impeachment of parents to be something of a lottery. They argued that there were no statutory means of protecting children before cases of parental cruelty were tried and no means of ensuring continued protection once convicted parents had served their sentences.[1]

The following steps were taken to remedy this situation. Inspectors, initially very few in number, were appointed to seek out and report to the police instances of abuse and neglect, even though until the passing of legislation in 1889 they had no legal authority or mandate to carry out this task. Shelters were established to provide places of safety for children pending prosecutions. They too were not backed by the force of law until later. Shocking cases of child mistreatment were publicized in order to influence public opinion and generate resources. Parliamentary lobbying to change the law regarding cruelty to children was relentlessly pursued. The outcome of all this pressure was the 1889 Prevention of Cruelty to Children Act. This Act defined specific parental misdemeanours against children and created penalties for wilful ill-treatment or neglect leading to unnecessary suffering or injury to health. It empowered police searches for children thought to be at risk, legalized removals to places of safety and enabled 'fit person' orders (the forerunners of care orders) to be imposed on children whose parents had been convicted of offences against them. Further Acts followed in 1894, 1904 and 1908, the effects of which were to consolidate and extend the original Act.

By this time the main components of child protection law that exist today were in place. As Dingwall *et al.* (1984) put it:

> there have been virtually no fundamental changes in the categories of children covered by the interventionist legislation since 1894. Subsequent legislation has consolidated the Victorian statutes and occasionally modernised their wording. It has introduced a few new types of disposition and redistributed enforcement duties. Nevertheless, the issues of principle were mostly settled in Victorian times.
>
> (Dingwall *et al.* 1984: 220)

The foundations were set even then for much of the form and style of current intervention practices in child protection work, according to

Ferguson (1990). In his lucid account of an NSPCC case in the north-east of England in 1898, he depicts an inspector grappling with the same contradictions and complexities as present-day social workers. Even at this early stage in child protection work, there was much emphasis on providing advice, support and material help. Much was being done to prevent court action as far as possible and to use it as a last resort. This style of intervention, which does not fit with the stereotype of the 'cruelty man', developed as a result of two main factors. First, NSPCC inspectors had to gain acceptance in commun-ities if they were to be effective. Second, their ultimate concern and that of the state was to inculcate a sense of responsibility in parents without totally undermining them. Prison and punishment were not seen as the best means of achieving this. Advice, persuasion and the threat of prosecution were methods that were more in tune with these twin goals.

By 1914 the NSPCC had established itself as a national institution. Its officers, together with its Scottish counterparts, covered the whole of the British Isles. Despite being feared in many communities, the NSPCC was also respected and this was reflected in the high percent-age of its referrals that came from neighbours and relatives. According to Behlmer (1982) 58 per cent of the 23,124 cases reported to the NSPCC in 1986–7 emanated from the general public.

Responding to sexual abuse

During this era, child sexual abuse within the family, previously ignored as an issue, was also being tackled by the NSPCC. Behlmer (1982: 70) notes that the London SPCC in its first year dealt with 95 cases involving 'domestic victims', of which 12 concerned 'an evil which is altogether too unmentionable' (sexual assault or incest). How-ever, despite this awareness and recognition, the NSPCC did not bring child sexual abuse to public attention in the same way as it had publicized physical abuse and neglect. This response reflected the gen-eral attitude to the issue, which was one of not wanting to know, a conspiracy of silence.

Child prostitution, by contrast, received far more public attention. In 1885, a journalist on the *Pall Mall Gazette*, William Stead, with the backing of influential social purity and child protection philanthrop-ists, wrote an exposé of a child prostitution ring that lured young English girls to brothels in Belgium. The series of articles he wrote were entitled 'The maiden tribute of modern Babylon' (see Bristow 1977; Gorham 1978). The outcome of these events was legislation to raise the age of lawful consent to intercourse for girls from 13 to 16, a response that Gorham (1978) views as inappropriate, but typical of the romanticized view of childhood held by middle-class Victorians, and also of their ignorance of the material conditions and pressures experienced by working-class female children.

The issue of intrafamilial abuse or incest meanwhile continued to receive little public attention or recognition. Where it was acknowledged, it was seen as linked to low intelligence and as a product of the overcrowded sleeping conditions of the poorer classes (Wohl 1978). Gordon (1989), drawing on the case records of the Massachusetts Society for the Protection of Cruelty to Children between 1880 and 1910, draws the same conclusion from the American experience:

> The NSPCC's ability to recognize incest, if not discuss it publicly, was in part based on its notion that it was exclusively a vice of the poor. Conservative and progressive reformers spoke of the degradation of poverty, as if its victims were animalistic, lacking in standards of family life.
>
> (Gordon 1989: 215)

Another popular explanation of this otherwise inexplicable vice was the demon drink.

There were, however, some public developments. The NSPCC, along with the National Vigilance Association, which had been formed in 1885, pressed for a law to criminalize incest, which was not a specific category of crime at this time. This pressure resulted in the passing of the 1908 Incest Act. Although the impact of this Act was very limited, at least incest was officially recognized as a crime and this in turn created the potential for more effective intervention given the will to intercede.

Protecting children within the family

As can be seen, there were considerable shifts in thinking about state intervention into family life between 1870 and 1914. I have focused on the child protection aspects, but one could look at a range of other areas, such as education, working conditions and health, and see similar developments taking place. However, child protection was a particularly problematic enterprise because it was at the most intrusive end of the process, in that it called into question parental behaviour inside the family home.

The responsibility of carrying out this task was taken up by religiously inspired philanthropic societies, most notably the NSPCC. Their workers faced the dilemma that social agencies still face: how, following liberal traditions, to influence the family without undermining its independence. That agencies did not wish to undermine families at this period is clear from the accounts of Behlmer (1982) and Gordon (1989): 'Under trying and occasionally hazardous conditions, therefore, cruelty men tried to stir a sense of parental duty in the adults they cautioned' (Behlmer 1982: 167). 'The SPCCs aimed as much to rein-force failing parental/paternal authority as to limit it' (Gordon 1989: 56). The goal was to change the internal behaviour of the family in order to ensure child protection, but without disrupting the order of things. Similarities between the late Victorian approach and that of the present response to child abuse abound.

Between the two world wars

A shift in focus

In contrast to the amount of change and degree of concern that characterized child protection work, particularly in the first three dec-ades of the 1870–1914 period, there was a definite shift in focus away from this issue between the two world wars. Early on in this period there was a sense that a corner had been turned. The 1923 Home Office report on the work of the Children's Branch pointed out that, despite the fact that the 1908 Children Act had broadened the grounds for neglect proceedings, the number of prosecutions of parents had dropped from 4106 in 1900 to 2052 by 1921 (Home Office 1923). The work of the NSPCC reflected these changes. In 1913–14 the NSPCC dealt with 54,772 cases. However, the number of prosecutions result-ing from these investigations was only 2349 (approximately 4 per cent compared with a prosecution rate of 10 per cent in 1895–6). Why had this shift in emphasis taken place?

Several reasons have been put forward. The 1923 Home Office report attributed the change to improved standards of parenting:

> The children of the poorer classes are better cared for than they used to be, and it is now unusual to see dirty and ragged children in the streets of our great cities. Cases of extreme brutality which were all too common not so many years ago are now becoming less frequent.
>
> (Home Office 1923: 69–70)

These improved parenting standards were seen to be the result of better welfare provision (for example school meals, health and child maternity services), changes in working-class habits (such as reduced alcohol consumption) and the work of agencies like the NSPCC. Rose (1991) attributed the perceived reduction in child abuse to the decline in the birth rate. He pointed out that the average number of children born to families in 1915 was 2.5 compared with 6 in the 1860s, and commented: 'One may conclude, therefore, that children being born from the Edwardian period were more "expected" and therefore on the whole more wanted than before' (Rose 1991: 243). Behlmer (1982) considered that two factors were at play. First, the First World War and the Depression diverted attention from the issue. Second, complacency had set in as a result of undue faith in the powers of the NSPCC to deal with the problem.

Dingwall *et al.* (1984) argued that child protection in itself had never been a major concern of the state, except in the 1880–1900 period. Its real worry was the threat provided by inadequate moral socialization of children to the social order. Neglect was seen as a cause of delinquency and was, therefore, considered to be an important target of intervention for that reason, not because of concern for the well-being of individual children.[2] Employing the work of Donzelot (1980), Dingwall *et al.* (1984) contested that throughout the first half of the twentieth century, the state recoiled from the direct attack on the family (and particularly patriarchal authority) that had taken place in the period immediately before this and redirected its efforts to bringing about change by means of support services focused particularly on mothers.

Gordon (1989), drawing from the North American scene, argued that the amount and type of child abuse did not, as far as she could judge, differ significantly during the whole period between 1880 and 1960. All that differed was the response to it. She linked societal concerns about child abuse and other forms of family violence to the strength of feminist thinking, arguing that when women have a strong voice, as they had in the late Victorian and early Edwardian eras, the effect of their pressure is to create a tougher response to the issue (though she hastened to add that this does not mean that the agencies established to deal with the problem share a feminist analysis of the problem). Her explanation, therefore, of the lack of overt focus on child abuse in the Depression period in the USA is as follows:

> One of the major characteristics of depression-era social work was a policy of defending the 'conventional' nuclear family ... A sympathy arose for the unemployed husband, the stress and role-conflict that frequently engendered his violence; remarkably less sympathy was mustered for the situation of mothers doing double shifts – at home and at work – in attempts to hold the family together ... Indeed violence altogether was deemphasised, and the SPCCs devoted themselves almost exclusively to child neglect, now conceived primarily in terms of economic neglect, such as malnutrition or inadequate medical care.
>
> (Gordon 1989: 22–3)

Apart from the fact that it is highly unlikely that between the two world wars British NSPCC inspectors delved into social psychological causes of male violence within families, this argument seems to have as good an explanatory value for the British situation as for that in the USA at this time.

All the foregoing explanations have some validity. There is no way of knowing for certain whether the incidence of child abuse during this era reduced or not. If socio-economic factors are taken into account, then despite the recession of the 1930s living standards were higher than in the late Victorian period and the extent of gross material deprivation was probably much less. These factors point to the likelihood of less abuse taking place, as reflected in official figures. However, it is also clear that there was a much less evangelical approach to the problem than in the previous era and a probability that a good deal of abuse went unnoticed.

Sexual abuse

Gordon (1989) provided one of the few accounts of official responses to child sexual abuse during this period. The case records that she studied showed that such abuse persisted throughout the whole period of her study (that is from 1880 to 1960). The 1880–1910 records showed that the SPCC workers of that time more readily accepted allegations of sexual abuse and that they judged child sexual abusers as socially and morally inferior beings. From 1910 onwards there was a much less direct, much more tentative approach to this issue, with far greater emphasis on abuse by strangers and on girls' sexual delinquency. In addition there was a good deal of victim-blaming. The problem of child sexual abuse, as Gordon (1989) saw it, though never high on the agenda, went underground for much of this time.

In Britain it is hard to find much reference to the subject. Prosecutions under the 1908 Incest Act remained at a low level, reaching 100 a year by the beginning of the Second World War. However, it is clear that some types of child sexual abuse were vigorously pursued at this time, judging from NSPCC accounts such as that by Housden (1955).[3]

The period 1945–70 and the rise of the children's departments

The Curtis Committee

There was an upsurge of interest in the welfare of deprived children after the Second World War. The report of the Curtis Committee (1946), which was set up to inquire into the conditions of children 'deprived of a normal home life with their own parents and relatives'

(1946: 5), provided a comprehensive and thoughtful account of the child care concerns of the day. However, it is notable that child neglect is referred to only briefly, and seems to win attention more because of its link with subsequent delinquent behaviour than for any direct concern about harm to the child (see note 2). This is despite the fact that one of the catalysts in highlighting the sorry condition of children cared for by the state at this time was the manslaughter by his foster-father of a 12-year-old child in care, Dennis O'Neill, a case that was being separately inquired into at the same time as the Curtis Committee was sitting (Home Office 1945).

The 1948 Children Act and its implementation

The 1948 Children Act was greatly influenced by the findings of the Curtis Committee and paid little attention specifically to child abuse. In the period following its implementation, however, there were some significant developments on the child abuse front.

In 1950 a joint circular was issued to local authorities, proposing the setting up of coordinating committees for overseeing 'problem family' cases that were being visited by a wide range of departments (Home Office 1950). Children's officers were appointed to act as chairpersons of these committees. Under the 1952 Children and Young Persons (Amendment) Act, children's departments' powers to intervene in cases where children were thought to need care and protection were broadened. This Act also empowered authorities to seek fit person orders on children without the requirement that parents first be prosecuted for cruelty or neglect. This change was seen to be beneficial in two ways. It enabled authorities to protect children more easily and it further reduced the need to prosecute parents, which was in tune with the less punitive approach towards families that characterized this period.

The other major development at this time was the push for a preventive approach to children and family work. This notion was attractive to a wide variety of constituencies. Child care officers, as a result of their direct work with families, saw that admissions to care were preventable given sufficient inputs of counselling and support before a crisis point was reached. Central government departments, concerned by a dramatic rise in the number of children in care immediately following the implementation of the 1948 Act, saw it as a cost-effective option. In addition they were concerned about the link between neglect and delinquency and the need to do something about the latter. There was also research support for a change of emphasis. Bowlby's study of institutional care for children and his resulting theories about the deleterious effects of maternal deprivation were prominent in this respect (Bowlby 1951; Bowlby *et al.* 1965).

Packman (1975) demonstrated how in practice throughout the 1950s child care officers had spent more and more of their time working with families to prevent receptions into care:

> By the 1960s, children supervised in their own homes far out-numbered those 'in care' and departments were involved, not only with a significant minority of all families with children (one-third of a million children, referred in one year, represents roughly 3 per cent of the total child population) but with a whole range of other services on their behalf.
>
> (Packman 1975: 72)

Such work received legal backing with the passing of the 1963 Children and Young Persons Act, section 1 of which empowered local authorities to provide material and financial assistance to keep children in their own homes where it was thought to be in their best interests.

Child care concerns in the 1960s

The main concern in the child care field for the remainder of the 1960s continued to be delinquency, the cause of which was seen to be neglect, and the solution, increased support for the family. The 1969 Children and Young Persons Act reflected this concern and analysis of the situation. Neglected children were treated by the law in the same way as children beyond control, children in moral danger, children refusing to go to school and children committing offences. As will be seen, when in the mid-1970s attention switched more directly to the ill-treatment of children by their parents, this legislation proved to be inadequate in many respects.

With regard to the professional response, there was a move towards a less specialized approach to child care work and to a broader family problem perspective (see Donnison 1954). Deprived children were seen to be the products of deprived families and a family-based service was considered to be needed, with a broader remit and more powers than before. Influenced by this type of thinking, the Seebohm report of 1968 recommended the formation of new unified social services departments comprising the former health and welfare and children's departments. These new departments were to be set up to 'meet the social needs of individuals, families, and communities' (Seebohm 1968: 43). These recommendations were made law and implemented in 1971.

Summary

On the face of it, the period between 1945 and 1970 was one in which family policy in general and the response to neglectful families in particular was relatively benign. As an extract from the 1960 Ingleby report shows, the policy style of the time was unequivocally family-oriented and family-sympathetic:

> In dealing with the prevention of neglect in the home, it is, in our opinion, essential to distinguish the following three stages:
> (a) the detection of the families at risk
> (b) the investigation and diagnosis of the particular problem
> (c) treatment: the provision of facilities and services to meet the families' needs and to reduce the stresses and dangers that they face.
>
> (Ingleby 1960: sec. 38, 17)

It is notable that it is families that are defined as being at risk and it is families that are expected to be the recipients of the treatment. Whether such a policy served the interests of the children and women in these families is an open question.

Once again, Gordon's (1989) account of the US situation is instructive, given the dearth of British studies of child protection during this period. She characterized the 1940–60 period as follows:

> The defend-the-conventional-family policy in social work continued through the 1940s and 1950s. These decades represented the low point in public awareness of family-violence problems and in the status of child protection work within the social-work profession.
>
> (Gordon 1989: 23)

She described an increasing psychoanalysation of family violence by social workers. In Britain, the influence of psychoanalytical theory on social work practice has always been much less than in the USA (see Yelloly 1980). Nevertheless, there can be little doubt that the work of Bowlby and the concerns about delinquency helped to focus attention on the emotional qualities of mothering and motherhood and emphasized the need to bolster families with advice, support and casework. Far less direct attention was paid to violence to children and to women within those families.

Sexual abuse, as we now perceive it, seems to have been even further from social workers' minds; the main forms of perceived sexual abuse at this time were either incest, seen as a rare and pathological phenomenon, or girls in moral danger because of insufficient controls being exerted by their parents (see Greenland 1958; Allen and Morton 1961).

Thus from a feminist perspective, policy responses to child abuse during this period were deficient in terms of protecting women and children from male violence. However, this period has been viewed by

other commentators as one of some enlightenment with regard to
child care issues rather than one of lack of vigilance. For instance,
Parton (1985) and Holman (1988) both consider the child protection practices of the period that will be reviewed in the next section
to be retrogressive and over-intrusive into family life in comparison
with this one, and they are critical of the decline in state support for
the family and the loss of emphasis on preventive work. As we shall
see, by the mid-1990s, after two decades of child protective thinking,
there was a shift back towards a family supportive approach very
similar in essence to that which characterized the 1950s and 1960s in
particular.

The rediscovery of child abuse 1970–85

Henry Kempe and baby battering

In the USA child abuse was formally rediscovered in 1962. In that year
Henry Kempe, a paediatrician, and his associates coined the term 'the
battered child syndrome', which described and explained the process
that led to parents (but essentially mothers) physically assaulting their
babies and young children (Kempe et al. 1962). Pfohl (1977) demonstrated that the first medical specialism to rediscover the problem was
actually that of paediatric radiology. However, Kempe and his colleagues were the first confidently to attribute injuries seen on children
to deliberate mistreatment rather than to the outcome of accident or
disease. Kempe argued that abuse of children was far more widespread
than anyone had previously considered and that professionals (doctors in particular) had been turning a blind eye to it. Kempe's original
thinking stressed the psychological aspects of child abuse. Essentially
his view was that child abuse resulted from emotional or psychological problems within the parents (or parent), which in turn stemmed
from their own emotionally depriving experiences in childhood. He
argued that parents needed psychological treatment or therapy, that
their children needed temporary protection and that in most cases
rehabilitation should be the goal. The main exceptions to this rule
were parents diagnosed as having psychotic illnesses. (For a fuller
account see Chapter 8.)

This model of child abuse was remarkably influential throughout
the USA in the 1970s and 1980s. Thanks to the tireless campaigning
of Kempe and others in this field, physical abuse of children became a
major social issue, attracting national publicity and massive funding
(see Nelson 1984). As early as 1967, every state in the USA had mandatory reporting laws and the Children's Bureau was spending considerable amounts of money on research into the problem.

It is hard to pinpoint the reasons for the re-emergence of this age-old problem in this new form at this time. Certainly, technological developments, such as the use of X-rays, played a part. However, Pfohl (1977) attributed much to the professional aspirations of paediatricians, who in an era of better physical health were in search of a new role for themselves. Neither explanation seems sufficient to account for the magnitude or persistence of the response to the issue. Broader social factors need to be taken into account as well. The climate was right for a greater focus on the care and upbringing of children. The relative affluence of the 1960s created the conditions for people to pay greater attention to the psychological needs of children and to the quality of parent–child relationships. Kempe's ideas were in tune with the times in that the notion of parents abusing their children as a result of a psychological syndrome was more acceptable than attributing such cruelty to poverty or ignorance. By giving child abuse a medical label and seeing it as a treatable condition, the new forms of intervention into family life were not seen as a threat to the independence of families in general because they were aimed only at the families that had 'the illness'.

The re-emergence of child abuse as a problem in Britain

Parton (1979, 1981, 1985) provided a detailed account of the development of child abuse as a social problem in Britain in the late 1960s and the 1970s. The pattern of development is similar to (and indeed greatly influenced by) that in the USA. He saw the growth of the problem as very closely linked to professional aspirations and to the politics of the family and the state.

There were two main professional groupings involved in the 1960s: medical doctors (most notably paediatricians) and the NSPCC. In 1963, Griffiths and Moynihan, two orthopaedic surgeons, used the term 'battered baby syndrome' in an influential article in the *British Medical Journal.* The amount of medical literature devoted to this topic developed steadily throughout the 1960s but the problem was not responded to at a wider level at this stage.

The NSPCC was facing an identity crisis at this time. Throughout the 1950s and 1960s, the new children's departments grew in size and stature and there was considerable overlap between their responsibilities and those of the NSPCC. Both were tackling similar problems in similar ways, but the children's departments were better resourced and had a broader statutory mandate. The emergence of a direct focus on physical child mistreatment, well established by the late 1960s in the USA, offered the NSPCC the opportunity of developing a more specialist and separate role. Contact was made with Henry Kempe and his associates, who were refining their ideas and developing new practice initiatives in Denver, Colorado. As a result, a project was established in London to provide specialist casework help for families referred for child abuse at a centre named Denver House. The work of this project was described and analysed by Baher *et al.* (1976). During this period the NSPCC was prolific in its publications on the subject of child abuse and was highly influential in placing it firmly on the social problem agenda (see Parton 1985).

Maria Colwell

What finally settled matters was the Maria Colwell case (Department of Health and Social Security (DHSS) 1974). Maria, aged 7, was killed by her stepfather in 1973. She had been in care for five years following a period of general neglect and low standards of care, and for nearly all of this time she had been boarded out with her aunt. Her mother had meanwhile remarried and had given birth to three children. In 1971, she was determined to have Maria back home. East Sussex County Council, in whose care Maria was, agreed to a plan of rehabilitation, supported Maria's mother's application to discharge the care order and recommended that it be replaced by a supervision order. Maria, who had been very resistant to returning to her mother, died 13 months later, grossly under-nourished and severely beaten by her stepfather. This was despite the fact that throughout this period there had been many health and welfare workers involved in the oversight of her development who had failed to 'see' the neglect and ill-treatment that she must have been subjected to over some considerable part of this time.

How the Maria Colwell case came to have such an impact was carefully analysed by Parton (1979). He argued that her death did not immediately cause a great deal of national concern. The key factor was the decision of the then minister of the Department of Health and Social Security, Sir Keith Joseph, to hold a public inquiry into what happened. Parton pinpointed the influence of a group called the Tunbridge Wells Study Group, consisting of paediatricians, lawyers and social workers, as a key factor acting on Joseph to make his decision. Joseph himself was very much in tune with the ideas of this group, as he was promulgating a more general thesis about cycles of deprivation among poor families and the need for such families to be targeted for specialist intervention (Joseph 1972).

The resulting inquiry, aided by media reports, especially in *The Times* and *Sunday Times,* arrested the attention of the public. Diane Lees, Maria's social worker, was vilified. The social work profession was considered to be too soft and permissive. The more benign family approach to child neglect issues, which had been prevalent since 1948, was thrown into question.

The establishment of a system for dealing with child abuse

As a consequence of the Maria Colwell inquiry report, the DHSS, by means of a series of circulars and letters, established the foundations of the system that currently exists for protecting children. The aims of the changes were to raise awareness of child abuse, to ensure that any allegation of abuse was promptly responded to, to improve interagency cooperation and to put in place more thorough systems for monitoring children considered to be at risk. The mechanisms for achieving these aims were:

- area review committees, consisting of higher and middle managers from all agencies with a role to play in the protection of children, whose function was to coordinate and oversee all work in this area
- case conferences involving all front-line professionals, whose function was to assess new cases and to review ongoing casework
- registers of all children considered to be abused or at risk of abuse.

Intervention into families with children considered to be at risk thus became, at least in form, more focused and intrusive. The concerns of the previous era, that is avoidance of separation of parents and children and support of and influence on the family as a whole, were now being officially called into question. The 1975 Children Act, which was largely concerned with more general child care issues, reflected the mood of the times. In particular, drawing on a study of long-term children in care (Rowe and Lambert 1973), it emphasized the needs of children as distinct from the rights of the parents. On the child protection front this Act made two major changes. First, it incorporated among the grounds for care proceedings the fact that a child was or might be living in the same household as a person who had committed offences under schedule 1 of the 1933 Children and Young Persons Act (that is offences of violence and indecency towards children). This was a direct result of the death of a child, Susan Auckland, at the hands of her father, who had previously been convicted for the manslaughter of another of his children (DHSS 1975). Second, it required the appointment of guardians *ad litem* to act exclusively on behalf of the child in cases like Maria Colwell's, when parents were seeking to discharge orders and the local authority was not opposing such courses of action. These changes reflect the fact that the new emphasis on abuse of children was already finding the 1969 Children and Young Persons Act deficient for the purpose of protecting them.

Child abuse work 1975–85

For the remainder of the 1970s the pressure to create a more effective detection, investigation and monitoring system for child abuse continued unabated. From 1973 to 1981 there were 27 inquiries into the deaths and serious abuse of children in Britain caused by their carers. In almost all these cases, various health and welfare agencies were already involved, often in a statutory capacity (see DHSS 1982). Mainly by means of advice and circulars from the DHSS, considerable effort was made to incorporate lessons from these inquiries into the structure of practice. From relatively small beginnings, child abuse work developed into a major preoccupation of social services departments.

The definition of child abuse broadened over time. This is well demonstrated by the changes in terminology. By 1980, the term 'child abuse' had replaced 'baby battering' and the subsequent term 'non-accidental injury'. The 1980 DHSS circular entitled *Child Abuse: Central Register Systems* outlined four categories of abuse or risk of abuse: physical injury; physical neglect; failure to thrive incorporated with emotional abuse; and living in the same household as someone convicted of offences under schedule 1 of the 1933 Children and Young Persons Act. At this time it is notable that sexual abuse of children was not considered to be a category for registration. This issue, already being addressed on a broad front in the USA, was only beginning to emerge as a social problem in Britain (see pp. 42–3).

In the first half of the 1980s there was some relaxation in the drive to establish better systems for responding to child abuse. There were fewer public inquiries (six in the three years from the beginning of 1982 to the end of 1984) and there was generally a consolidation of the rash of changes that had taken place in the 1970s. By this time, social services departments were firmly in the lead role in this field, despite official concern to emphasize the inter-professional aspects of the work.

Intrusive social work practice?

Between 1970 and 1985 state intervention into families to protect children had certainly become more systematic, in the literal sense of the word. Whether it had become more intrusive into families is open to question. The most comprehensive research into practice during this period was that of Dingwall *et al.* (1983). They argued that the 'new' response to child abuse was tougher in aspect than in practice. They tried to demonstrate that, despite greater concerns for children at risk, social workers, by and large, were still operating in a relatively benign way with families (similar to the pre-Colwell era). They identified what they described as a 'rule of optimism' in action, whereby social workers were expected to make the best interpretation of an allegation of abuse. This 'rule', they argued, was not one of social workers' own making, but reflected prevailing liberal democratic views about the respective roles of the state and the family with regard to the upbringing of children: namely that while the state has a legitimate role to play in intervening into families to ensure the protection of children, this should be done only with due regard to the rights of parents as well as to the assessed needs of children. Thus the liberal approach that they identified being adopted by social workers was in general terms in line with the requirements of the state.

Parton (1985) cited the increase in the use of place of safety orders in the 1970s and of the gross numbers of children in care as evidence of a more intrusive approach towards families. His view of the situation is as follows:

> It would thus appear that social work practice with children and families has become far more authoritative and decisive and has increasingly come to intervene in ways which can be experienced by threats or punishments.
>
> (Parton 1985: 127)

Corby (1987) found from a study of early intervention into families suspected of abusing their children that the form and style of this intervention was, from the parents' viewpoint, punitive and severe. Parents suspected of abusing their children were at first treated with great suspicion, were poorly informed of what was happening and had no rights of attendance at case conferences. However, after the initial stages of intervention, this highly proceduralized and apparently punitive approach gave way to a more sympathetic and helpful response in many cases. Relatively few cases resulted in court action and there was evidence to support Dingwall *et al.*'s (1983) view that, overall, intervention was characterized by a cautious optimism.

Arguably, therefore, it can be concluded that increased state intrusion into family life between 1975 and 1985, while being officially encouraged, was in practice being tentatively implemented. The focus was still on working with families as far as possible.

Jasmine Beckford, Cleveland and the 1989 Children Act 1985–91

Developments in the general child care field

At the same time that social workers were being encouraged to take a firmer stance on child abuse, there were counter concerns being put forward about the dangers of over-intrusive, heavy-handed practice in the general child care field. Parton (1991) dated these concerns from 1978.

First, a series of studies was commissioned by the DHSS, resulting in a number of publications summarized in a report entitled *Social Work Decisions in Child Care* (DHSS 1985a). These studies, while not directly focused on child abuse, came to the general conclusion that not enough attention was being paid to the needs of families in child care work. In particular, some were critical of what they saw as the overuse of compulsory powers (Packman 1986).

Second, the House of Commons Social Services Committee chaired by Renee Short undertook an inquiry into children in care and reported in 1984 (House of Commons 1984). Parton (1991: 27–39) gives a good summary and analysis of the working and findings of this committee. It took as its major concern the perennial problem of the relationship between the state, children and the family, namely how the state can best ensure the protection and welfare of children and provide support for the family in achieving this goal without undermining its independence. In particular it was vexed by the relative weight to be given to professional discretionary powers (especially those of social workers) and to a legally enforced rights-based approach, and came to the conclusion that there should be a shift towards the latter. Place of safety orders and parental rights resolutions were particular instances of concern. The report recommended the establishment of a working party on child care law, whose report in 1985 (DHSS 1985b) laid the foundation for the 1989 Children Act.

The Jasmine Beckford inquiry

On the child protection front there was a major development, though in a totally different direction from that being taken in the broader child care field. The year 1985 saw the publication of the Jasmine Beckford inquiry report (Brent 1985). Jasmine, aged 4, died in July 1984, emaciated and horrifically beaten over an extended period of time by her stepfather, Morris Beckford. Jasmine and her younger sister, Louise, had both suffered severe injuries in 1981, for which Morris Beckford was given a suspended sentence. The children were committed to the care of Brent Borough Council and lived with foster-parents for six months. They were then returned to their parents, who had been helped with rehousing and had been allocated a family aide, on a home-on-trial basis. The social services department supported the family somewhat spasmodically over the next two years. Jasmine was seen only once by the social worker in her last ten months of life. This social worker, Gunn Wahlstrom, was described by the judge at the trial of Morris Beckford and Jasmine's mother as being 'naive beyond belief' and was subjected to the same sort of negative publicity that Diane Lees had been exposed to eleven years earlier.

The inquiry report made 68 recommendations. Its main concerns were that social workers were too optimistic with regard to the families with which they were working. Dingwall et al.'s (1983) 'rule of optimism' was mistakenly interpreted to support this view. The report stressed that too much emphasis was placed on the rehabilitation of Jasmine and her sister to their parents, and that, in the process, evidence to suggest the likelihood of further abuse was ignored. Further, it emphasized that although other agencies were to blame to some extent for what happened, the main fault lay with Brent Social Services Department because it was legally *in loco parentis* with regard to Jasmine by virtue of the care order made in 1981. The report was unequivocal in its view that social work's essential and primary task was to protect children and that where necessary social workers should employ the full force of the law to ensure this.

The findings of the Beckford inquiry had an immediate impact on policy and practice. The DHSS (1986) published draft guidelines setting out recommendations for improving inter-professional coordination in child abuse work and inviting comments. The main proposed changes consisted of reframing child abuse work as child protection work, thus emphasizing the statutory obligation placed on local authorities to act primarily on behalf of children wherever risk was perceived. It was proposed that area review committees be re-termed joint child abuse committees (but in the final guidelines issued in 1988 they were in fact renamed area child protection committees) and that child abuse registers become child protection registers. The key role of social services department workers was again reaffirmed and strengthened. They were allocated the main responsibility to coordinate work (now called a protection plan) with families whose children's names had been added to the child protection register. Among the other changes, it is notable that with regard to parental participation at case conferences, a topic that had been concerning a wide range of professionals and pressure groups (Brown and Waters 1985), the recommendation was that it was not appropriate for parents to attend formal case conferences, although they could attend informal meetings with key professionals who were involved with them. The tone and message of this document were identical to those of the Beckford inquiry report (Brent 1985) – the focus of attention was to be shifted to the protection of children first and to consideration of the needs and rights of parents second.

The effects of the Beckford inquiry report seem to have been immediate. Statistics regarding child protection registers (see Chapter 6) show a massive rise in the numbers of children being placed on them after 1985. The number of place of safety orders increased dramatically in 1986 and 1987 after nine years at roughly the same level, and there was a significant rise in the number of children coming into care as a result of child abuse and neglect.

The Beckford report was followed by a series of other inquiries into child deaths. Between 1985 and 1989 there were 12 such inquiries in all, the findings of which are summarized in a study of inquiry reports during 1980–9 (Department of Health 1991a). What all the physical abuse inquiries of this period were at pains to emphasize was the need for a child-focused approach, with much more emphasis on assessing families for potential risk.

Child sexual abuse

The counter-concern for a greater family-focused approach coming from those concerned with the general problems of children in care was augmented from an unlikely source. In the summer of 1987, newspapers reported a child sexual abuse scandal in Cleveland. It emerged that 121 children had, over a period of six months, but mostly in the two months of May and June, been brought into care on place of safety orders on the recommendation of two paediatricians who, using a physical test pioneered in Leeds, had diagnosed the majority of them as having been anally abused. The parents of these children were in uproar and had attracted the attention of the local Labour MP, Stuart Bell, to their cause. He raised the matter in Parliament and the outcome was the establishment of another, but this time very different, public inquiry.

Up to this time the issue of child sexual abuse had been a relatively minor concern for child protection agencies in Britain. However, a good deal of pioneering work had already been carried out before events in Cleveland in a quieter and less controversial way. As with physical abuse, concerns about the sexual abuse of children originally stemmed from experience in the USA. The main protagonists there were survivors of sexual abuse (Armstrong 1978; Brady 1979; Angelou 1984), feminist writers such as Rush (1980) who saw such abuse as symptomatic of gender power inequalities, and the medical profession. Among the latter, Kempe and his associates were again prominent (Kempe and Kempe 1978). Another approach to the problem was developed by Giaretto et al. (1978) in California (see Chapter 10).

Giaretto's work was a major influence on the British approach to the problem developed by a team of child psychiatrists, psychologists and social workers at the Great Ormond Street Hospital for Sick Children (see Ben-Tovim et al. 1988; Furniss 1991). Their approach, which will also be considered in more detail in Chapters 8 and 10, was to develop a method of intervention based on family therapy principles. In addition they developed techniques (again pioneered in the USA) for helping children disclose the fact that they had been sexually abused, using drawings, play, anatomically correct dolls and video-recordings. These techniques were taken on by social workers in several statutory agencies and figured in events at Cleveland.

By 1987 child sexual abuse was beginning to clamber on to the official child protection agenda, though the response to the problem throughout Britain was patchy and variable. A MORI Poll survey commissioned by Channel 4 television had demonstrated that one in ten children had experienced some form of sexual abuse by the age of 15 and in half of these cases the abuse had been committed either by a family member or somebody known and previously trusted by the child (Baker and Duncan 1985). In Leeds a child sexual abuse ring had been discovered in the mid-1980s, involving children of a much younger age than had been previously thought to be associated with such abuse (Wild 1986). Paediatricians there developed the anal reflex dilatation test (Hobbs and Wynne 1986), which was seen as a break-through in terms of providing definite physical evidence of sexual abuse, which up to this time had been almost impossible to prove in the courts.

The Cleveland affair

These developments set the scene for what happened in Cleveland. The rash of child sexual abuse diagnoses there and the subsequent removal of children into statutory care can be attributed to a combination of factors. First, there was heightened awareness of the possible extent of sexual abuse of children among key social services personnel and community paediatricians. Second, the paediatricians were aware of the newly developed reflex anal dilalation test, convinced of its validity and determined to use it. Third, other agencies, particularly the police and police surgeons, were more traditional in their approach and did not accept the new thinking, thus creating a major split in the inter-professional approach. Fourth, the social services department had recently reorganized its child protection system in response to the findings of the Beckford inquiry. The result of this cocktail of factors was that the paediatricians diagnosed far more cases of sexual abuse than had previously been the norm, the social services department acted swiftly and authoritatively to secure place of safety orders on all diagnosed cases and the police and police surgeons, who would usually have been closely involved in gathering evidence for possible prosecutions, dissociated themselves completely from what was happening.

As a result, large numbers of children were committed to care, many of whom were inappropriately placed for long periods in hospital wards because there were insufficient social services department facilities to cope with such an influx. Although all the children had been diagnosed as being abused, it was not clear who had abused them. Social workers, using the techniques developed by Ben-Tovim and his colleagues, were holding a series of disclosure interviews to try to establish facts, and in the meantime those parents who were potential suspects were being denied access to their children in order to ensure that they did not influence their evidence.

The main findings of the Cleveland inquiry report (Butler-Sloss 1988) resulting from these events confirmed that child sexual abuse was a more widespread phenomenon than had previously been thought to be the case. The chair of the inquiry, Lord Justice Elizabeth Butler-Sloss, was at pains to stress that, whatever criticism might be levelled at various practitioners, child sexual abuse must remain on the social policy agenda. The report also criticized individuals from every agency and profession for not working together more cooperatively. In particular, social workers were judged to have rushed in overzealously to rescue abused children (the opposite of the criticism levelled at them in most of the physical abuse inquiries). The report also recommended that greater consideration be given to the rights of parents (in terms of being fully informed of decisions) and to those of children, particularly with regard to medical examinations (because of the disagreements between professionals at Cleveland some children had been examined on four or more occasions).[4] Finally, it criticized the use of the reflex anal dilatation test without supporting social evidence.

These findings and recommendations had an almost immediate effect. The draft *Working Together* guidelines issued in 1986 were hastily amended to incorporate its recommendations (DHSS 1986, 1988). Some of the changes created a complete turn-round in policy, most notably that relating to parental participation at case conferences. Whereas the 1986 draft had stated that it was inappropriate for parents to attend, the 1988 view was as follows:

> They should be invited, where practicable, to attend part, or, if appropriate the whole, of case conferences unless in the view of the Chairman of the case conference their presence will preclude a full and proper consideration of the child's interest.
>
> (DHSS 1988: para. 5.45)

These guidelines placed greater emphasis on careful interdisciplinary consultation before intervention in sexual abuse cases and recommended joint police and social services department investigations to be the norm.

The 1989 Children Act

The Cleveland report also had an impact on the passage of the 1989 Children Act through Parliament. There were hasty amendments to the Act, such as that empowering children to refuse to undergo medical assessments if they so wished (sec. 44(7)) and that enabling local authorities to provide or pay for accommodation for alleged abusers so that children could remain at home during investigations (schedule

2 para. 5). This Act was already very much a mixed bag. The main thrust for change had come through the general concerns about children in care already documented and the need to improve the use of voluntary care to make it more supportive of families. Another influence had been the need to make the law more specifically responsive to child abuse cases and to avoid the use of wardship that had grown apace throughout the 1980s (see Lowe 1989). Another had been to give greater legal rights to parents and less discretionary power to professionals, for example with regard to contact with children in care and the use of emergency measures. Yet another aim had been that of consolidating all child care law, public and private, under one piece of legislation. Meanwhile public inquiries like Jasmine Beckford (Brent 1985), Kimberley Carlile (Greenwich 1987) and now Cleveland (Butler-Sloss 1988) continued to raise other issues and controversies. All the changes in the legislation that were emphasizing increased parental participation, more voluntaristic approaches and greater control over professional discretion by the courts were reinforced by events in Cleveland.

Concluding comments

There are a variety of reasons for the somewhat bewildering developments between the Jasmine Beckford inquiry report and the passing of the 1989 Children Act. They can best be understood by reference to the way in which the issue of child abuse was responded to in earlier years.

Throughout the whole of the period reviewed in this chapter, there was ambivalence and uncertainty about the best way for the state to intervene in families to ensure that children are properly socialized and not ill-treated, whatever the view about the motives for this concern. Preserving the independence of the family and the rights of parents has always had to be balanced against the welfare of children and their rights to be protected by those sanctioned by the state to carry out child protection work. For many years this task was left to the judgement of inspectors from the NSPCC and later to that of child care officers in children's departments, with backing from the courts as and when required. This approach was deemed to be working well as long as support for the family remained the major goal. The rediscovery of child abuse challenged this consensus position, just as it did in the late Victorian era. Social workers and other professional workers in this field were increasingly pressed to intervene more authoritatively into families in the light of the knowledge that abuse of children by their parents was more widespread than had previously been thought to be the case. They did this at first rather uneasily and were pressed further following the Beckford inquiry. However, those concerned with more general child care matters were of the view that social workers were being inappropriately intrusive into families where such an approach was not required, and lobbied for more legal rights for parents and more legal control over social workers.

A major turning-point came with the increased attention being paid to sexual abuse. The more zealous approach that had been encouraged by the state in the case of physical abuse was seen as inappropriate with regard to sexual abuse. Campbell (1988) has argued that the reason for this apparent about-turn is that the extent of child sexual abuse by males which events at Cleveland pointed to was seen as threatening to men, and the response was, therefore, to defend the family against what were seen as outrageous attacks from outside. While this interpretation may have some validity, it is clear that backing for a more family-supportive approach had already developed considerable momentum by the mid-1980s, as evidenced by the findings of the Short report (House of Commons 1984). Economic and broader social changes, as well as gender factors, have also played a part in these developments in the child protection field. The new softening which, as we shall see in Chapter 4, developed considerably in the 1990s may well be linked to concerns about the family under threat from recession and unemployment, high divorce rates and the growth of lone-parent families.

Whatever the explanation, there can be little doubt that the scene was set at the start of the 1990s for entry into a new stage of child protection work. There have been times when specific focus on child protection has been the main concern (the late Victorian era and 1970 to the present) and times when a broader family-supportive approach to child care issues has predominated (from 1914 through to the end of the 1960s). On the face of it, the 1989 Children Act pointed to greater emphasis being placed on family support again. However, events in the preceding 20 years created an awareness of the fact that families could be dangerous and distressing places for many children. Chapter 4 will look at how these conflicting demands and ways of thinking have impacted on child protection work to the end of the 1990s.

Child abuse: a historical time-line 1800–1990

1800–70   State concern with
            • children of the streets
            • children at work
            • young offenders
            • Poor Law children

1861	Offences Against the Person Act
1872	Baby farming
	Infant Life Protection Act
1887	Formation of the NSPCC
1889	Prevention of Cruelty to Children Act
1908	Children Act
	Incest Act
1933	Children and Young Persons Act
1945	Dennis O'Neill inquiry
1946	Curtis Committee
1948	Children Act and formation of children's departments
1950	Coordinating committees (cruelty and neglect)
1962	Henry Kempe and the battered child syndrome
1974	Maria Colwell inquiry (non-accidental injury)
	Formation of the child abuse prevention system
1975	Children Act
1974–80	Seventeen more public inquiries into child abuse deaths
1980	Broadening of concerns (child abuse)
1981–5	Fifteen more public inquiries into child abuse
1984	Short report
1985	Jasmine Beckford inquiry
	MORI Poll survey into child sexual abuse
1985–90	Fourteen more public inquiries into child deaths
1986	Draft *Working Together* guidelines (child protection)
1987	Kimberley Carlile and Tyra Henry inquiries
1988	Cleveland inquiry
	Working Together guidelines
1989	Children Act

Recommended reading

Behlmer, G. (1982) *Child Abuse and Moral Reform in England 1870–1908.* Stanford, CA: Stanford University Press.

Gordon, L. (1989) *Heroes of their Own Lives: The Politics and History of Family Violence, Boston 1880–1960.* London: Virago.

Hendrick, H. (1994) *Child Welfare: England 1872–1989.* London: Routledge.

Merrick, D. (1996) *Social Work and Child Abuse.* London: Routledge.

Parton, N. (1985) *The Politics of Child Abuse.* London: Macmillan.

Parton, N. (1991) *Governing the Family: Child Care, Child Protection and the State.* London: Macmillan.

Rose, L. (1991) *The Erosion of Childhood: Child Oppression in Britain 1860–1918.* London: Routledge.

chapter **four**

CHILD PROTECTION AND FAMILY SUPPORT IN THE 1990S

After the implementation of the Children Act in October 1991, social workers and other child protection professionals experienced great uncertainty about how to respond to child abuse concerns. As we saw in Chapter 3, whereas there had been a fairly uniform message sent out to social workers and other professionals with a child protection remit from the time of the Maria Colwell inquiry up to the publication of the Cleveland report, the messages post-Cleveland were very mixed. While there was no encouragement to relax vigilance particularly with respect to serious physical abuse, there was more emphasis on the need to adopt a cautious approach with regard to sexual abuse. The Cleveland inquiry was clearly a watershed. The image of the pro-family social worker failing to identify children at risk was replaced by that of the over-zealous interventionist who was prepared to stop at nothing to uncover family secrets. For many politicians, civil servants and social work academics, the excesses of Cleveland were clear evidence that the shift from the family support approach which had been prevalent from 1948 until the early 1970s had gone too far.

One of the first initiatives taken following Cleveland by the Department of Health was to set in train a series of research projects to examine the extent and consequences of different forms of child abuse and perhaps more significantly to look in detail at how various aspects of the child protection system operated in different geographical areas. The impact of these studies when they reported in 1995 was, as we shall see, of considerable significance.

Ritual/Satanist abuse

If Cleveland upset those concerned about over-zealous state intrusion into the family, events immediately after in relation to the investigation of what has been variously termed ritual, Satanic or Satanist abuse more than confirmed their views.[1] The late 1980s saw a rash of such investigations in Congleton, Rochdale, Manchester, Liverpool and Nottingham, to name but a few areas. The main features of these cases were accounts by young children of themselves and others being involved in rituals with adults (including often their parents and/or carers) dressed in cloaks and various black magic paraphernalia and being subjected to (or witnessing) acts of sexual indecency and physical cruelty. These allegations were mainly responded to by social workers and police with a series of interviews with the children following their removal to places of safety on emergency orders. These investigations aroused considerable publicity which early on was quite supportive of the child protection professionals. However, in most of the cases, this support quickly turned to criticism following adverse comments about the nature and quality of interventions made by judges faced with a lack of hard evidence in subsequent court hearings.

The Orkney case

Matters came to a head following a case in the Orkneys in 1991. During the course of interviewing a number of children from one family who were suspected of having been sexually abused by their father and siblings, allegations of ritualistic sexual abuse of nine children from four other families were made, implicating their parents and a local minister. These children were subsequently summarily removed from their homes in a joint police and social work manoeuvre, flown to mainland Scotland and placed in foster care where they were subjected to much interviewing and denied any contact with their parents. Six weeks later, a decision was reached at the sheriff's court that the legal proceedings that had taken place were incompetent and the return of the children to their parents was ordered.

The public inquiry that was subsequently held reported in 1992 (Clyde 1992). As with the Cleveland inquiry report, the Orkney report did not consider whether the alleged abuse had taken place or not, but proceeded to examine the reasonableness of the actions of the child protection professionals in the light of the information they had available to them. The inquiry panel was particularly concerned to examine whether the mode of treatment of children and their parents during the investigation was necessary. The overall findings of the Orkney inquiry were consistent with those of Cleveland. Lord Clyde was particularly critical of the style and quantity of the interviewing of children (it was considered to be insufficiently objective and far too frequent and intense), of the manner of the removal of the children from their homes (the dawn raid tactics employed were deemed unacceptable), and of the ban on contact between parents and children following their removal (it was considered to be traumatic for both and unnecessary for the protection of the children). The net outcome of this inquiry was to confirm the need for a less intrusive style of intervention into child abuse cases.

The spate of concerns about Satanist abuse disappeared almost as suddenly as it had started. The Department of Health, following the Orkney inquiry, commissioned research into all allegations of ritual abuse that had taken place from 1987 to 1992. The research conducted by Jean La Fontaine found that there was no hard evidence in any of the 84 cases that she considered to support the notion that there were Satanic cults carrying out rituals which involved the torture and killing of children. However, there was evidence of sexual abuse of children in a large number of these cases, sometimes by one perpetrator, but more often by more than one perpetrator either from within extended family networks or in a few instances by organized paedophile rings (La Fontaine 1994). Writing in 1998, La Fontaine explained the rise and fall of concerns about Satanist abuse as stemming from a combination of circumstances involving Christian fundamentalism, the influence of North American writing about such abuse in the early 1980s and the readiness of child protectionists in certain areas to believe literally what she clearly thought were the fantasies of disturbed and deprived children, many of whom were being subjected to appalling sexual (but not Satanist) abuse (see La Fontaine 1998). Compelling and persuasive though La Fontaine's account is, she could not refrain from attributing blame to social workers trying to disentangle some of the mystifying evidence with which they were faced;[2] it is notable that those who did believe that children were being sexually abused as part of Satanic rituals have since been vilified in the press (see Corby and Cox 1998).

Working Together *guidelines 1991*

In response to Cleveland and some of the earlier ritual abuse cases, new child protection guidelines were produced in 1991 outlining the needs for more measured, planned and coordinated interventions (DoH 1991b). In particular, it was made a requirement that social workers and the police should conduct joint investigations into all serious cases of physical abuse and into all allegations of sexual abuse. In 1992, guidelines were issued setting out in detail the requirements for videoed joint interviews, which, following the recommendations of the Pigot Committee, were to be allowed as evidence-in-chief at the criminal trials of alleged abusers in order to ease the pains for child witnesses in court (Home Office/Department of Health 1992). By these means, it was intended to prevent the 'excesses' that had been witnessed in the previous five years or so.

Institutional abuse

The 1990s saw a massive growth in concern about the abuse of children living away from home, particularly in regard to children in the care of the local authority. Linked to this, there was also concern about the abuse of children in nurseries. Between 1990 and 1996 there have been at least ten public inquiries into abuse in such settings, outstripping the number of inquiries of abuse of children in their own homes (see Corby *et al.* 1998). This is in stark contrast to the 1970s and 1980s when there were three inquiries into institutional abuse – in Lewisham (1985), Belfast (DHSS (Northern Ireland)

1985) and Greenwich (Social Services Inspectorate (SSI) 1988) – compared with nearly fifty into abuse by family members.

The Pindown inquiry

In 1991 a report was published about the use of a system called Pindown in children's homes in Staffordshire (Staffordshire 1991). This report outlined how in one area of the authority residential workers implemented a crude method of controlling children in care who were considered to be challenging in their behaviours. It was essentially a form of solitary confinement based very loosely on sensory deprivation principles. Children were kept in poorly furnished rooms for long periods, deprived of outdoor clothing, not spoken to by staff, and given tedious and repetitive tasks to complete. This system operated for over six years and had the tacit approval of the management of Staffordshire Social Services. Overall, 132 children came under the Pindown regime during the years in question. The youngest child thus treated was 9 years of age. One child was kept under this regime for a total of 84 continuous days. Not surprisingly, the inquiry found the Pindown regime to be abusive in the extreme.

Other inquiries into institutional abuse

In the period immediately following the publication of the Pindown report (Staffordshire 1991), a series of concerns were raised about regimes in Southwark, Brentwood, Bradford, Lincolnshire, Kirklees, North Wales, Islington, Sheffield, Lambeth and Chepstow. Inquiries had also been started in Leicestershire and in Gwent (South Wales). Here the concerns were about the sexual abuse of children in residential care. The Leicestershire inquiry reported in 1993 (Leicestershire 1993). Its primary focus was on the activities of the head of one of that authority's homes, Frank Beck, who had been convicted of a series of sexual and physical assaults on children in his care in 1991. Beck had gained something of a local reputation for using regressive therapy with adolescents, which involved them returning psychologically to babyhood and being treated and handled as though they were babies. With hindsight, it was apparent that Beck's grasp of the theory was crude and misguided; it served to enable him to further usurp his power over the children and young people in his care. The report condemned these activities, but perhaps more tellingly, was very critical of the general poor standards of accommodation provided for children and of the lack of vigilance by the management of Leicestershire Social Services Department.

The government's response

The Department of Health responded to this flurry of concern about abuse of children in care by commissioning its own more general inquiries into the state of residential care services for children in England (Utting 1991; Warner 1992). Similar inquiries took place in Scotland and Wales (SSI Wales 1991; Skinner 1992).

The Utting (1991) report provided a useful overview of the strengths and weaknesses of residential care at the time. It reaffirmed the low status of such care, the low level of qualified staff, the impact of a decline in the use of residential care, and the fact that it had become more and more a last resort choice of placement for children and young people with particular problems and difficulties. It asserted the need for maintaining a reasonable range of residential facilities and for more positive use of them, particularly in relation to young people. With regard to abuse, the report seemed satisfied that changes in the 1989 Children Act, particularly those relating to making representations (sec. 26), carrying out inspections and appointing visitors to children in care where necessary were sufficient to prevent the sort of ill-treatment that had been in evidence in Staffordshire.

The Warner Committee, which was set up as a direct result of the prosecutions of Frank Beck, was more focused on the recruitment of staff to residential care and advocated better training and more rigorous selection procedures, both of which recommendations were subsequently acted upon. Pay was another concern and was considered by the Howe (1992) Committee. In addition, the Department of Health set in train a series of research projects into different aspects of residential care which were eventually to be published in 1998 (DoH 1998a).

These initiatives, however, did not stem the flow of new concerns about abuse of children in residential settings. Allegations of sexual abuse and physical mistreatment of children resulted in inquiries about day nurseries in Newcastle (Hunt 1994) and at a residential boarding school for children with learning difficulties in Northumbria (Kilgallon 1995), and wide-scale police investigations into almost all children's homes in Merseyside, Cheshire, Clwyd and Gwynedd. In response to these increased concerns, the Department of Health commissioned a further inquiry into the situation of all children living away from home; this reported in 1997 (Utting 1997). In addition to children looked after by local authorities, this report took into account children spending long periods in hospitals, in all types of boarding schools and in foster care. The main message of the Utting report was to reaffirm the need for considerable vigilance, but it also stressed that measures were being put into place to ensure greater safety for children not living in their own homes.

A further response by central government was to concede to pressure from North Wales (Clwyd and Gwynedd), where it was being alleged that widespread sexual abuse had been taking place, possibly involving powerful figures and a large-scale cover-up, by setting up a tribunal of inquiry. This type of inquiry is the most formidable means of carrying out quasi-judicial investigations into matters of national concern and had never been previously used in connection with child abuse. The choice of this means to inquire into events in North Wales reflected the extent of concern that abuse of children in care generally had raised in society. This inquiry finally reported in 2000. It is as yet too soon to assess what influence it will have on residential child care policy and practice, though several factors suggest that it may not have the impact that was hoped for by those who pressed for it. First, the abuse being inquired into took place mainly before 1992 and extends as far back as 1974. Second, the Department of Health-sponsored research (referred to above) has been published, presenting a broad and comprehensive picture of key issues in residential care today (DoH 1998a). Third, practice initiatives are being developed through a programme entitled *Quality Protects* which specifically aims to tackle issues relating to health, educational and social issues in relation to children in care (DoH 1998b). Finally, in relation to the monitoring and inspection of care facilities, which local authorities currently carry out themselves, proposals have been made in the government White Paper, *Modernising Social Services* (DoH 1998c), to place the responsibility for such activities on more independent regional bodies.

Summary

To summarize, the 1990s saw an explosion of concern about the abuse of children in care. The extent and nature of this concern is interesting because much, though not all, of the abuse investigated during this period took place in the 1970s and 1980s. Statutory residential care is much diminished in size now by comparison, but (as we have seen) currently concern about the abuse of children has spread to a much wider range of out-of-home settings.

There seem to have been four types of abuse taking place in residential settings. Wardhaugh and Wilding (1993) have identified the two most obvious ones, those relating directly to the regime's measures of control, as in Pindown, usually involving psychologically cruel or physically abusive practices, and sexual abuse usually perpetrated by individual residential workers using the power opportunities provided by their positions in the homes, as in Leicestershire. A third form of abuse is linked to issues of neglect in situations where children are not contained within the residential centre, and become involved in unacceptable behaviours such as offending, drug-taking and prostitution. Concerns of this kind were raised in the Islington inquiry (White and Hart 1995). Most recently, there was an inquiry into the death of Aliyah Ismail (Harrow 1999), a 13-year-old girl in the care of Harrow Social Services Department. She died of a methadone overdose and was known by various child protection professionals to have been involved in prostitution. The last form of abuse relates to bullying by peers within institutions. Sinclair and Gibbs (1998) found that this was a widespread concern among children in care whom they interviewed.

Organized abuse, paedophiles and child prostitution

As we saw in the section on Satanist abuse, much of the ritual abuse investigated by La Fontaine (1998) could be described as organized by virtue of the fact that there was more than one abuser involved and in some instances more than one abused child. However, the extent of the organization she found was very variable. A good deal of the abuse of this nature took place within extended families and may have been linked to the culture and prevailing power relationships within those families.

The popular image of organized abuse is that of paedophile rings in which children are systematically passed round to be sexually abused or to be coerced into the production of pornographic material (or both). Such abuse may not be entirely extrafamilial as it may well commence via family connections and follow on from intrafamilial abuse. Paedophile rings are also associated with child murder – the Jason Swift case is a classical example of this type of abuse.[3] Paedophile rings are also often considered to be in operation in institutional abuse, particularly where more than one child abuser has been convicted in one home. It is worth noting, however, that, as yet, no evidence of the operation of such rings has been found in these settings. The main pattern of abuse seems to be that of one perpetrator operating alone and in secrecy, but often abusing more than one child.

The existence of paedophile rings is not in question, but the extent of them is. Bibby (1996) estimated a national incidence rate of organized abuse as a whole to be 278 cases a year. Only a small proportion of these cases will involve organized extrafamilial rings. The notion of a large network of evil people preying on vulnerable children outside the family can, therefore, be dispelled.

However, the public perception and fear of 'the paedophile', whether operating in rings or alone, whether abusing positions of responsibility to gain access to children or picking them up in parks or on the streets, has remained strong in the public mind, and led to important

changes in policy and practice during the 1990s. The main developments are in relation to the movements of offenders released from
prison and to the tightening up of systems of criminal checks for
those seeking employment involving contact with children. The
degree of concern about paedophiles has been such that in some areas
their addresses have been published in newspapers and there have
been residents' protests as a result. While some of these responses are
understandable, they do have dysfunctional outcomes. In relation to
institutional abuse, it is argued that emphasis on deviant individuals
infiltrating themselves into a vulnerable institution diverts attention
away from the shortcomings of the actual institutions (Stanley 1999).
Another dysfunction of the demonization of paedophiles is that not
enough work is done to understand their ways of thinking or to
differentiate between types of paedophile activities and motives for
abuse (see Colton and Vanstone 1996; Featherstone and Lancaster
1997).

Finally, in this section, brief consideration will be given to the issue
of child prostitution which has been the cause of much concern in
the late 1990s. Important work has been carried out by voluntary
agencies to develop better understanding of how girls in particular
become prostitutes emphasizing how they can be entrapped and later
coerced into such activity against their will. As a consequence of this
research, it is proposed in the new *Working Together* guidelines (DoH
2000a) that such children should not be viewed as offenders, but as
victims of abuse.

Intrafamilial child abuse: the resurrection of family support

All the foregoing developments in the 1990s were largely in relation
to abuse that takes place outside the family or on the fringe of the
family. In this section we pick up the story with regard to physical
abuse, neglect and sexual abuse within the family.

As stressed at the beginning of this chapter, the early 1990s saw
social workers operating with a much greater degree of uncertainty
than before. In the first two years after the implementation of the
1989 Children Act, the numbers of care proceedings and applications
for emergency care orders reduced considerably. There was a fair degree
of tentativeness in pursuing allegations of sexual abuse within the
family (see Corby 1998). Greater attempts were made to work more
closely with families in this period. Parental participation at conferences became more common, as did professional–parental con-
sultations in the period following initial interventions. While there
were those that queried the nature of this more partnership-focused

approach (Corby *et al.* 1996), it cannot be denied that the impact of the Children Act and the then new *Working Together* guidelines (DoH 1991b) were having some loosening up impact.

Messages from research 1995

In 1995, the research projects set up by the Department of Health following the Cleveland inquiry report were published individually (20 in all). They were also summarized in *Child Protection: Messages from Research* (DoH 1995) and implications for child protection policy and practice were distilled from their findings.

The main findings of these research projects were as follows.

1 The child protection system acted like a giant sieve taking in a broad spectrum of referrals about the care of children, ranging from concerns about the demeanour of toddlers in nurseries through to allegations of incest. In all, 24 per cent of these referrals resulted in child protection conferences and at just over half of these, recommendations were made for placement on the child protection register (see Gibbons *et al.* 1995a).

2 Most of the 85 per cent of families not registered received minimal intervention and service provision. Services were centred on children and their families who had been placed on the child protection register (Gibbons *et al.* 1995a).

3 However, nearly all families that were subject to initial child protection investigations were poor, had experienced considerable problems, such as death, divorces, accidents and illnesses (physical and mental) and had previously been referred or were current service users. The children in most of these families were in need (Farmer and Owen 1995).

4 Parents at the receiving end of child protection investigations experienced them as difficult and stigmatic forms of intervention. Many parents felt that they were being unfairly labelled as child abusers. To their mind, child abuse was equated with serious physical assaults and sexual abuse, not with problems with parenting (Farmer and Owen 1995).

5 There were too few attempts to engage parents in the child protection process either by giving adequate information or by enabling participation at child protection conferences. There was little evidence of working in partnership with parents (Thoburn *et al.* 1995).

6 In terms of child protection, there was overall a 70 per cent success rate, using incidence of reabuse as an indicator.

The general picture was that the child protection system had become too bureaucratized, too proceduralized and over-focused on overt incidents of child abuse, such as bruising or sexual abuse allegations. As a consequence of this, broader family problems and, in particular, the issue of general neglect, were tending to be overlooked. If more obvious forms of abuse were not present, then the likelihood was that families would receive little attention from child protection professionals, even though a broader assessment might have identified the existence of many unmet needs as far as the children in these families were concerned. The summarizing document, *Child Protection: Messages from Research* (DoH 1995) also made great play of the fact that research of the kind carried out by Egeland *et al.* (1983) indicated that children living in generally neglectful situations suffered worse long-term consequences in terms of personal, social and economic development and success than the majority of those who were physically and sexually abused. The point being made was that standards of care in neglectful families tended to persist throughout childhood whereas other forms of abuse might be isolated or spasmodic. The emphasis was on the psychological impact of such abuse. It was deemed that children living in persistently adverse conditions, while possibly experiencing the most psychologically damaging effects, were the least likely to receive supportive services.

What was needed, therefore, in child protection work was a shift in both resources and thinking about working with families. Child protection professionals needed to be less concerned with externally identified abuse and more focused on tackling the psychological impact of being a child in need. In practical terms, this might mean redefining much that had previously been considered to fall under the label of child abuse and treating it in a qualitatively different way from more overt and potentially damaging forms of ill-treatment in the short term. By redefining many of what were previously termed child protection referrals as concerns about children in need, and by redefining the process of engagement as assessing children in need (as opposed to carrying out child protection investigations), the aim should be not only to reduce stigma but also to direct more resources to meeting the needs identified. Revisions of the *Working Together* guidelines (DoH 1991b) and of the 1988 assessment tools (DoH 1988) were finalized early in 2000 (DoH 2000a, 2000b) reflecting these shifts in thinking. There is far greater emphasis in these documents on working in partnership than previously and considerable concern to ensure broad-based assessments and interventions. Child abuse is seen as one of a series of concerns about families that might be referred, not necessarily the focal one in all cases. Indeed, both documents seem to be very wary of using the term child abuse at all, so far has the shift in thinking progressed.

While the move back towards a more family supportive approach commenced under a Conservative administration, it is noticeable that under the current Labour government, the emphasis has changed somewhat, in that there is now a clearer acceptance of the extent of child poverty in Britain (or of socially excluded children, if you like) and of the need to make a concerted effort to diminish it. The effect has been to broaden the debate and at the same time to add impetus to the shift towards family support. The focus is now on general child welfare rather than on the safeguarding of children, though it is stressed that the two are not incompatible. The outcome of the new developments remains to be seen.

Countervailing views

This shift in thinking has not been an entirely smooth one, and there is still much disquiet as to whether the current proposals are realistic and as to whether they will enable child care/child protection professionals to achieve the right sort of balance between support and protection.

There are those who consider that the true extent of child abuse has still not been fully recognized, and that, therefore, it is premature to think of taking the pressure off child protection professionals involved in tackling such abuse. The NSPCC commissioned a survey in 1994 and in the report that resulted from this, it was estimated that 1 million children could be defined as being abused in Britain (NSPCC 1996).

Those who have looked more closely at the issue of dealing with sexual abuse of children within families have raised questions as to how, in the current climate, it is possible to combine working in a family supportive way with protecting children in such cases (Masson 1997; Corby 1998).

There is particular concern that a shift to a more family supportive approach may mean that children are placed at greater risk of physical abuse and neglect. This message has been driven home hard again by the NSPCC in its current Campaign to End Cruelty to Children, which highlights the number of fatal abuse cases that have taken place during the 1980s and 1990s (NSPCC 1999). The Bridge (1998), a child care consultancy service, has also been heavily involved in pointing out the dangers of a less than vigilant approach in dealing with child abuse and neglect. This agency was very active in the 1990s in carrying out Part 8 Reviews for area child protection committees where children had been seriously and fatally abused.[4] Several of these reviews have been made public, most notably those relating to a child called Sukina in the area of Avon, a child named Paul who died as a result of neglect by his parents in Islington, and the West children in Gloucestershire (Bridge 1991, 1995a, 1995b). This experience has convinced the Bridge's director and staff of the need for much greater attention to be paid to careful recording and checking of danger signs by professionals; it has promoted its own assessment schedule (Bridge 1997) which is in marked contrast to that being officially promoted by the Department of Health, in that its focus is much more centred on the notion of the dangerous parent, drawing on knowledge of circumstances in which children have died as a result of abuse.

There is a sense among agencies such as the NSPCC and the Bridge that there is insufficient openness about serious abuse because focusing on it seems to fly in the face of the more positive approach to working with children and families that the present Labour administration is at pains to promote.

There is also concern about whether there are sufficient resources being allocated to enable the new developments with their broader remit to work effectively. The shift to providing more family support for those families referred for child protection concerns has considerable resource implications, both in terms of person power, because of the greater emphasis on assessment of all referred cases, and in terms of the services required as a result of the outcomes of those new assessments (see Tunstill 1997). There is no doubt that the previous Conservative government was greatly concerned with the increasing costs of the child protection system: the report of the Audit Commission (1994) pointed out that child protection was taking the lion's share of child care budgets within local authorities. This problem has been very evident in the USA as well, where it is estimated that 3 million child protection referrals are being made annually (Elders 1999). Clearly, economics had some part to play in the debate about shifting the focus from child protection to family support, being fuelled to some degree by the expectation that it would be at least partly financed by a reduction in the child protection system's administration costs. However, with the broadening of the debate on to aspects of more general social exclusion, this does not seem to be feasible. The issue of costs does not seem to have been fully addressed.

Finally, there has also been some disquiet among child protection professionals about the new shift as well. There has been some concern about the research that laid the foundation for the changes currently under way. It has been argued that there was very little emphasis placed on the professional viewpoint in this research (Parton 1996). Much more emphasis was placed on the consumer view, that is that of the parents and the children. Given events in Cleveland which were the catalyst for this research, this was understandable, and in many ways admirable, in that the perspective of service users had been rarely considered at all in previous years. Nevertheless, there was a sense that the research did not explore as fully as it might have why professionals were operating in the way that they were, whether the more authoritative approach that the parents reported was a preferred style, and what the resource constraints were. It could be argued, for instance, that social services departments in particular were deliberately allocating scarce resources to the highest priority cases. It could also have been argued, with some considerable justification, that the focus on child protection which had been adopted was very much in line with the demands of the public over the previous 15 or so years, and that, therefore, the criticism was unjustified.

Concluding comments

The 1990s saw a major transformation in thinking about and responding to child abuse in Britain. The post-Cleveland concerns about over-intrusion into families dominated the early part of the decade. Fuelled further by social work's incursion into the controversial field of Satanist abuse, and by increasing societal concern with abuse of children in residential care and the emergence of the paedophile, the focus gradually shifted away from intrafamilial child abuse. In 1995, the publication of *Messages from Research* (DoH 1995) proved a major turning-point in this respect; the second half of the decade saw a consolidation of the shift that took place in the first half. Things have moved so far that the term child abuse now seems to be used with great caution. While the Department of Health is determined not to be accused of ignoring the problem, there can be little doubt that in its eagerness to move towards a more family supportive approach that fits in with broader policy developments in relation to the family and the issue of social exclusion, intrafamilial abuse has been relegated to a position of much less prominence than before. This shift has not been without criticism, and no doubt any new child abuse tragedies might well be attributed, particularly by its opponents, to the evolution of the family support policy.

It is notable that Britain seems to be undergoing this shift in isolation. Many other countries in Europe already operate family supportive policies in relation to child protection issues. However, most of these countries have maintained these policies throughout and have not gone through the changes that have taken place in Britain (see Pringle 1998). Indeed some countries consider the systems that Britain has developed to be well in advance of their own, which stem from more traditional non-interference in family affairs approaches. In the USA there has been a crisis in confidence in child protection similar to that which has been experienced in the UK. This has been particularly driven by the sheer pressure of numbers of referrals rather than by other concerns. One of the key responses in the USA has been to place much greater emphasis on risk assessment strategies in order to be able to concentrate resources more closely on those children deemed as a result to be most at risk.

There are many ways of construing reasons for the direction that events have taken place in Britain since 1990. As identified in Chapter 3, there has been tension for a considerable time between two schools of thought about how best to ensure the protection of children within families. There are those who have been in favour of more positive pro-family measures as an indirect means of meeting the needs of children at risk, and there have been those who have argued for more direct child protective measures (see Fox-Harding 1991). The former are now in the ascendancy partly as a result of economic arguments (that is the high cost of the child protection system), partly as a result of the support of those who see the need for the family to be protected from outside interference, and more latterly, as a result of the emphasis currently being given to the tackling of social exclusion.

That such a shift should have taken place is to some degree apparently against the trend to reduce risk in society which has been identified by some writers as an explanation for the increased concern about child abuse since the 1960s (Parton *et al.* 1996; Munro 1999). However, it could be argued that the new strategy does not represent a lessening of concerns about risk to children within the family, but, rather, a bold move towards a more preventive approach to child abuse.

Key events in child protection in the 1990s

1991   • Implementation of the 1989 Children Act
        • Publication of new *Working Together* guidelines
        • Report of the inquiry into the Pindown regime operating in Staffordshire
        • Utting report into the state of residential care for children
        • Sukina inquiry report

1992   • Orkney inquiry report
        • Publication of the *Memorandum of Good Practice* providing guidance for interviewing of children for evidence in child protection cases

- Warner report into the selection, training and management of staff for posts in residential care for children
- Howe report into salary for staff in residential care settings

1993
- Report of the inquiry into the abuse of children in Leicestershire children's homes

1994
- Report into the abuse of children in nurseries in Newcastle upon Tyne
- La Fontaine report on ritual abuse
- Report of the Audit Commisssion

1995
- *Paul: Death from Neglect* report
- Report into the abuse of children with learning difficulties in a residential school in Northumbria
- Inquiry into the management of children's residential services in Islington
- Publication of *Messages from Research*
- Report on the child abuse aspects of the West case

1996
- Commencement of the North Wales tribunal of inquiry
- Report of the NSPCC commission of inquiry

1997
- Utting safeguards review report

1998
- Publication of *Residential Care: Messages from Research*
- Government proposals: Quality Protects, Modernizing Social Services

1999
- Report into the death of Aliyah Ismail

2000
- New *Working Together* guidelines and assessment framework

Recommended reading

Corby, B. (1998) *Managing Child Sexual Abuse Cases*. London: Jessica Kingsley.
Department of Health (1995) *Child Protection: Messages from Research*. London: HMSO.
La Fontaine, J. (1998) *Speak of the Devil: Tales of Satanic Abuse in Contemporary England*. Cambridge: Cambridge University Press.
Parton, N. (ed.) (1997) *Child Protection and Family Support: Tensions, Contradictions and Possibilities*. London: Routledge.

Parton, N., Thorpe, D. and Wattam, C. (1996) *Child Protection, Risk and the Moral Order*. London: Macmillan.

Utting, Sir W. (1997) *People Like Us: The Report of the Review of the Safeguards for Children Living Away from Home*. London: HMSO.

chapter **five**

DEFINING CHILD ABUSE

Clearly any logical approach to a problem entails describing its nature and size, so that the response to it can be appropriate and sufficiently well resourced to ensure an effective solution. However, as we saw in Chapters 3 and 4, child abuse is not a phenomenon that lends itself easily to logical solutions because of its political, cultural and historical underpinnings. Child abuse is a highly complex issue and, as will become evident, is not easily defined or measured. Although the two topics are closely interrelated, since the way in which abuse is defined influences its extent, for the purposes of analysis they will be considered separately. This chapter will critically consider issues relating to the definition of child abuse and Chapter 6 will be concerned with measuring its extent.

Defining child abuse

Before we look at different categories of child abuse, some general considerations should be taken into account.

The cultural context of child abuse definition

Child abuse is a socially defined construct. It is a product of a particular culture and context and not an absolute unchanging phenomenon. As we saw in the historical survey, what is considered to be abusive in a particular society alters over time. Place is another factor. Anthropological studies show clearly that what is viewed as abusive in one society today is not necessarily seen as such in another, Korbin (1981) cites examples of culturally approved of practices in societies in the southern hemisphere that we would almost certainly define as abusive:

> These include extremely hot baths, designed to inculcate culturally valued traits; punishments, such as severe beatings, to impress the child with the necessity of adherence to cultural rules; and harsh initiation rites that include genital operations, deprivation of food and sleep, and induced bleeding and vomiting.
>
> (Korbin 1981: 4)

She points out that the reverse is also true:

> Practices such as isolating infants and small children in rooms or
> beds of their own at night, making them wait for readily available
> food until a schedule dictates that they can satisfy their hunger,
> or allowing them to cry without immediately attending to their
> needs or desires would be at odds with the child-rearing philoso-
> phies of most of the cultures discussed.
>
> (Korbin 1981: 4)

The lesson to be learned from anthropological studies is that the
cultural context within which behaviour takes place and the meaning
attributed to it by those sharing that culture are important factors to
be taken into account when labelling certain acts as abusive.

Although such comparisons rightly sensitize us to the culturally
relative nature of child abuse, this does not mean that there can be no
common standards at all. Korbin (1981) stresses that the sort of abuse
described by Kempe *et al.* (1962) as the 'battered child syndrome'
would not be sanctioned by any society. Finkelhor and Korbin (1988)
argue that there are some culturally approved practices, such as ritual
circumcision and clitoridectomy, that should be universally seen as
abusive and addressed as such.

The issue of sensitivity to culture applies within societies as well as
between them. However, just the same sort of care needs to be taken
with a culturally relativist approach in these circumstances. Dingwall
et al. (1983) were of the opinion that the standards applied by social
workers observed in their study ran the risk of being too low. They
were so used to dealing with poor families and poor parenting skills
that they accepted them as the norm for that culture. Stubbs (1989)
showed how misguided assumptions about cultural differences between white social workers and Asian families can lead to a failure to
protect children in these families from abuse. Such views are borne
out by some of the public inquiry cases and go some way to explaining the extraordinary degree of tolerance shown by social workers in
cases like that of Stephanie Fox (Wandsworth 1990), Lester Chapman
(Berkshire 1979), Paul (Bridge 1995a) and Tyra Henry (Lambeth 1987).[1]
Differentiating between culturally normative and abusive or neglectful parenting is a critically difficult but essential task for child protection social workers.

The concerns of the definers

Another general issue relates to the formal definitions of different
types of child abuse. There are a bewildering number of such definitions emanating from a wide range of sources. It is important to know
who the definers are, and what are their aims, goals and interests. For

instance, Henry Kempe *et al.* (1962), in their original definition, deliberately used the emotive term 'battered child' because they wished to draw public attention to the issue. Their definition of the phenomenon and account of its causation reflect a clinician's concern with the individual: 'a clinical condition in young children who have received serious physical abuse generally from a parent or foster-parent' (Kempe *et al.* 1962: 17) Contrast this definition with that of Gil (1975), a sociologist, with clear views about the broader political aspects of the treatment of children. He defines child abuse as 'inflicted gaps or deficits between circumstances of living which would facilitate the optimal development of children to which they should be entitled and their actual circumstances, irrespective of the sources or agents of the deficit' (Gil 1975: 346–7).

These two definitions are poles apart. Were one to take action according to the latter, all the 4 million children living in or 'on the margins' of poverty in Britain (Kumar 1993) would probably be on child protection registers. Kempe and Helfer's (1962) definition, on the other hand, would limit the numbers to those identified by health and welfare agencies as being physically abused or exposed to physical abuse by their parents.

Legislators, by and large, favour non-specific definitions of abuse because they allow flexibility and room for manoeuvre. Therefore, most legal definitions of child abuse are phrased in very general terms, such as 'improper treatment' or 'significant harm'. In the USA in the early 1980s there was a reaction against such general definitions on the grounds that they encouraged unwarranted and harmful interventions. Wald (1982) proposed that the legal definition of physical abuse be limited to 'injuries inflicted on a child which cause or create a substantial risk of death, disfigurement or impairment of bodily functioning'. While such a definition achieves the goal of specificity, many might find it unacceptably narrow as a basis for deciding upon intervention. However, recently in Britain, both researchers (Thorpe 1994) and those responsible for policy developments (DoH 1995) have been critical of child abuse interventions for being based on definitions that are too broad (see also Gough 1996).

Researchers into child abuse are very much concerned with achieving precision and consistency. Clear identification of the object of research and common standards of measurement are important ingredients of such work. As we shall see in the section on prevalence (pp. 96–7), inconsistencies of definition between studies may well account for major differences in findings (Finkelhor and Baron 1986). Besharov (1981) considered that definitional inadequacy has had harmful effects on research:

There are thousands of different and conflicting definitions of 'child abuse' and 'child neglect' in use today. Some describe child

maltreatment in terms of proscribed parental conduct; some focus
on the harm to the child; and many are couched in both. While
many definitions share common approaches, elements, and even
phraseology, the different combinations and permutations seem
endless.

(Besharov 1981: 384)

Defining child abuse in practice

A further general issue relates to the process by which child abuse is
actually defined in practice. Here we are considering what Gelles (1982)
termed operational as opposed to nominal definitions (that is those
used in law and research). How do social workers and other professional groups in fact decide what does and does not constitute abuse
from the large number of referrals they receive?

Giovannoni and Becerra (1979) were of the opinion that there were
no adequate definitions of abuse that could be operationalized by
professionals: 'A major thesis of this book is that child abuse and
neglect are matters of social definition and that the problems that
inhere in the establishment of those definitions ultimately rest on
value decisions' (Giovannoni and Becerra 1979: 5). To test this hypothesis, they devised 78 pairs of vignettes briefly describing potentially
abusive situations.[2] Half the vignettes outlined the consequence of
the potential abuse; half did not. The researchers assigned 60 vignettes
at random to four groups of professionals (police, social workers, paediatricians and lawyers) and to non-professional inhabitants of Los
Angeles, who were asked to rate them on a 1 to 9 scale of seriousness.

The main finding was that there was little agreement between the
professional groupings about the seriousness of the various types of
abuse. Overall, there was most agreement between the police and
social workers, who together took a more serious view of nearly all
incidents than did the paediatricians and lawyers (in that order). This
lack of agreement was attributed to the requirements of occupational
roles. Thus the reason for higher ratings on the part of police and
social workers was seen to be their greater involvement in the early
investigative stages of abuse. The police rated vignettes where a crime
had been alleged as more serious than the other professionals. Social
workers were ahead of the others with regard to emotional abuse and
lawyers tended to rate everything lower than the rest because their
concern was whether there was enough evidence to prove a case in a
court of law.

With regard to non-professional people, Giovannoni and Becerra
(1979) found that as a whole they were more likely to judge the
scenarios as more serious than all the professionals and that those
from the lower social classes 'generally saw mistreatment as more

serious than did those of higher socioeconomic status' (Giovannoni and Beccera 1979: 189). This is in contrast to the widely held perception that professionals have higher standards in this respect than the general public (see Christopherson 1983). The main conclusion drawn from Giovannoni and Becerra's study was that there was much confusion among professionals over deciding whether cases were sufficiently abusive to justify intervention. Examination of cases dealt with in one geographical area showed that this confusion carried over into practice and that there was a good deal of inconsistency with regard to decisions. Smaller-scale studies in Britain have come to similar conclusions (Corby 1987; Higginson 1992). Giovannoni and Becerra (1979) advocated the abandonment of the general terms 'child abuse' and 'neglect' and recommended replacing them with more precise legal definitions of the various categories.

On the basis of these studies, the only safe definition of child abuse is that it is a judgement reached by a group of professionals on the examination of the circumstances of a child, normally (in Britain) at a child protection conference. Such a definition is usually symbolized by placing the child's name on a child protection register.

In Britain, central government in its 1995 review of DoH-sponsored research programmes has accepted the view that child abuse is socially constructed (DoH 1995). It concludes that the best way to understand the mistreatment of children is by viewing parental handling of children as a continuum ranging from the acceptable/desirable through to the seriously abusive. It argues that professionals, acting on behalf of society (and presumably reflecting its views) determine the threshold of abuse and that this can shift over time. It suggests that the threshold currently operating in Britain is relatively low compared with preceding eras and that there is a need to reconsider some of the concerns that have driven this development. It is argued that more attention needs to be paid to the impact of different styles of intervention and to the long-term consequences of different situations before defining them as child abuse. The exposition of ideas such as these by a government department clearly exemplifies the social and political aspects of defining child abuse.

Formal definitions of child abuse

In Britain, formal definitions of child abuse derive from Department of Health guidelines and these will be used as a framework for the rest of this section. There are also legal definitions to be found in section 31 of the 1989 Children Act.[3] In addition, new types of abuse and concerns not covered by these definitions are emerging and these too will be considered.

The term 'child abuse' was first officially used in Britain in a 1980 government circular (DHSS 1980). As described in Chapter 3, four categories of abuse were specified: physical abuse; physical neglect; failure to thrive and emotional abuse (a combined category); and 'children living in a household with, or which is regularly visited by, a parent or another person who has abused a child and are considered at risk'. Where identified, such children's names were to be placed on a register. Prior to this, there had been no specific definitions used by central government. By 1988, there were five categories of child abuse: physical abuse; neglect; emotional abuse; sexual abuse; and grave concern (DHSS 1988). By 1991, the categories had been reduced to four again, grave concern having been eliminated (DoH 1991b). These four categories have been retained in the 2000 guidelines, but redefined (DoH 2000a).

Physical abuse

Physical abuse was the original concern of the child protection lobby and in the public mind was synonymous with child abuse until the publicity surrounding intervention into child sexual abuse cases in Cleveland in 1987. In the 1999 guidelines, physical abuse is defined as involving

> hitting, shaking, throwing, poisoning, burning or scalding, drowning, suffocating, or otherwise causing physical harm to a child. Physical harm may also be caused when a parent or carer feigns the symptoms of, or deliberately causes ill-health to a child. This situation is commonly described using terms such as fictitious illness by proxy or 'Munchausen syndrome by proxy.'
>
> (DoH 2000a: 5)

As a nominal definition, this categorization is more specific than before. However, it is not particularly useful as an operational definition because there is little guidance as to when any of these behaviours becomes serious enough to warrant protective intervention. The only guidance in this respect comes from the concept of significant harm in the 1989 Children Act which is the type of vague and general definition of the kind that (as we have noted above) legislators tend to approve. Wald's (1982) definition (see p. 68) is much more focused and prescriptive but, as stressed before, probably too restricted in scope. In practice, there are many factors taken into account in deciding whether officially to define a situation as abusive (that is by registration).

Seriousness

The seriousness of the injury plays a part. Minor bruising, for instance, though frequently cited as a precursor to more serious abuse,[4] is generally not seen as sufficiently serious to require registration, even where there is suspicion that it has been non-accidentally inflicted. A series of unexplained bruises, on the other hand, is more likely, under the same circumstances, to be considered sufficient cause for such action. Serious physical maltreatment in suspicious circumstances is normally defined as unequivocally abusive.

Intention

Intention has generally been considered to be a key variable in deciding whether an action is abusive or not (though it is not one specified in the 2000 guidelines). Again there is variation with regard to this. Dingwall *et al.* (1983), in their study of child protection systems, identified among some hospital doctors what they termed a strict liability approach (Dingwall *et al.* 1983: 36). From this point of view, if a child suffers a serious injury even accidentally, the child's carer at the time should accept responsibility for the outcome and can be judged to be abusive. For the majority of child protection workers, however, intentionality is seen as an influential factor. It would be unlikely, for example, for children accidentally injured during a fight between their parents to be registered on the grounds of physical abuse. However, the violence in the household and its psychological impact on the child would be a cause for concern and possible registration, depending on the context, under the category of emotional abuse (see pp. 80–1).

Age of child

A factor often taken into consideration in defining physical abuse is the age of the child. Generally, the younger the child suspected of being physically abused, the greater the likelihood of official registration. This response is frequently justified by the fact that young children (particularly those under school age) are physically more vulnerable and less open to being monitored by health and welfare professionals. Physical abuse of older children can also sometimes be seen to be an over-zealous use of physical punishment that, while disapproved of, is considered understandable within a culture that supports some forms of physical correction (see Freeman 1988). Such an explanation is less acceptable in the case of very young children.

Context and risk

The context in which physical mistreatment abuse takes place is another important factor in deciding whether or not to define it as abusive. Current government guidelines (DoH 2000a), in line with the more recently developed approach to child abuse outlined in Chapter

4, are at pains to stress the importance of taking contextual factors into account when making decisions about whether to treat a case as one of child abuse, for example family strengths and weaknesses, the child's general health and development, the child's reaction to the incident concerned and the adequacy of parental care.

The concern with context is linked to some degree to the notion of risk assessment which is again an important part of the defining process. In most cases once the immediate consequences of abuse have been dealt with and a reasonable degree of immediate safety for the child established, the focus shifts from the actual incident and injury to consideration of the risk to the child in future. The Department of Health has published new assessment guidelines and procedures (DoH 2000b) which are required to be carried out in all cases where child abuse is considered following referral to be a major concern. These guidelines are broad-based and have a concern to balance child protection with family support. There are other forms of risk assessment which are less concerned with the general future needs of the child, but focus specifically on the risk of further abuse (see Greenland 1987; Bridge 1998). The various forms of assessment are dealt with in more detail in Chapter 10. However, it is worth noting here that the latter approach to assessing risk of abuse to children has been the subject of considerable criticism both in Britain and in the USA (see Corby 1996), and in the current climate in Britain, the use of checklists as predictors of physical abuse is likely to diminish in the immediate future.

Evidence for court

A final issue in relation to defining physical abuse is that of proving physical abuse in court. The standard of proof obviously has to be higher for care proceedings than for deciding whether or not to place a child's name on the child protection register. Medical evidence is the key factor. X-ray material, blood-clotting tests and expert opinion are the main sources of evidence. Paediatricians have largely been cautious in their assessment of cases of physical abuse and have thereby gained credibility in courts. There are still controversial issues, the most notable of which is whether brittle bone disease might be the cause of some symptoms diagnosed as being the outcome of abuse (see Carty 1988; Paterson and McAllion 1989).

Reasonable chastisement?

A key question for courts in some cases is whether inflicting physical harm is justifiable because it results from punishment used to discipline a child, that is, is it reasonable chastisement? As we have seen, the younger the child the less acceptable it is to use physical force to achieve compliance. With older children, there is generally far more tolerance. This was challenged in 1998 in the case of a 9-year-old boy who was beaten by his stepfather with a garden cane. A charge was brought against the stepfather and dismissed in the English court. The case was then taken to the European Court of Human Rights where it was found that the judgment was not in accordance with the rights of the child. As a consequence the British government is intending to pass legislation which will clarify what forms of physical punishment are acceptable or not, presumably by defining where a child may be hit and with what. This case and government reaction to it has led to a campaign to ban parental use of physical punishment totally and thereby to bring English law in line with eight other European countries which took this step in the 1980s and 1990s (see Freeman 1999). Much evidence has been produced to demonstrate the adverse consequences of such punishment (see Leach 1999). This has been countered by those who see smacking as not only harmless but positively beneficial. The outcome of this debate may not be seen for a few years, but there is little doubt that greater clarity about the issue of acceptable physical punishment will ultimately be welcomed by child protection workers.

A note on Munchausen syndrome by proxy

The official definition of physical abuse includes poisoning, suffocation and Munchausen's syndrome by proxy (see p. 71). These are relatively rare forms of abuse. The fact that they are highlighted probably reflects the fact that they often result in fatalities or other serious outcomes. The deliberate administration of harmful substances was included in Kempe's early descriptions of child abuse (Kempe and Kempe 1978). The issue of suffocation has received a good deal of publicity because some doctors (Meadow 1989; Newlands and Emery 1991) believe that up to 10 per cent of cot deaths may be the result of this form of abuse.[5] Such a viewpoint has been condemned by others because there is no clear-cut evidence for such a belief and the suggestion is thought to be highly insensitive to relatives of cot death children (see letters in the *British Medical Journal* (1989) vol. 299, pp. 178–9 and 455–6).

There is a growing body of medical literature about Munchausen's syndrome by proxy (see Meadow 1977, 1985; Mehl *et al.* 1990; Bools *et al.* 1994). First diagnosed in 1977, the syndrome is characterized by a child presenting with an illness that has been fictitiously produced by a parent, typically the mother. The child is subjected to abuse by exposure to the medical treatment prescribed. Meadow (1985) was aware of 90 cases in Britain. More recently, the term 'illness induction syndrome' has been suggested as a replacement for the term 'Munchausen syndrome by proxy' (see Gray and Ben-Tovim 1996). It is seen as a less esoteric title and also as one which can incorporate a range of abuses (including suffocation and poisoning) which have a common causal base, that is parental psychological or emotional disturbance.

Physical neglect

Neglect is defined in the Department of Health 1999 draft guidelines as:

> The persistent failure to meet a child's physical and/or psychological needs, likely to result in the serious impairment of the child's health or development. It may involve a parent or carer failing to provide adequate food, shelter and clothing, failing to protect a child from physical harm or danger, or the failure to ensure access to appropriate medical care or treatment. It may also include neglect of, or unresponsiveness to a child's basic emotional needs.
>
> (DoH 2000a: 6)

As with the definition of physical abuse, this definition of neglect is more specific than that found in the 1991 guidelines (DoH 1991b). However, as an operational definition, it is still problematic. Practitioners must determine what counts as 'persistent failure' and 'serious impairment'. They must also be able to define basic psychological and emotional needs.

Definitions drawn from the American scene are more specific:

> It is presumed that physical, emotional and intellectual growth and welfare are being jeopardized when, for example, the child is:
>
> 1 malnourished, ill-clad, dirty, without proper shelter or sleeping arrangements;
> 2 without supervision, unattended;
> 3 ill and lacking essential medical care;
> 4 denied normal experiences that produce feelings of being loved, wanted, secure and worthy (emotional neglect);
> 5 failing to attend school regularly;
> 6 exploited, overworked;
> 7 emotionally disturbed due to constant friction within the home, marital discord, mentally ill parents;
> 8 exposed to unwholesome and demoralizing circumstances.
>
> (Polansky et al. 1972: 4–5)

This definition is at least more specific about those areas of care (or lack of it) to which attention should be drawn, but the question of standards is still not resolved. For instance, how ill-clad and dirty does a child have to be to be defined as neglected? At what age can a child be left unsupervised? Terms such as 'exploited', 'emotionally disturbed' and 'unwholesome and demoralising circumstances', far from clarifying matters, pose even more definitional problems.

Cultural relativity

An additional problem is that there is no consideration in Polansky *et al.*'s (1972) definition of issues such as cultural relativity, material resources and intellectual capacity, which are all important considerations for operational definitions of neglect. Stevenson (1998) considers these issues, that is whether we can distinguish between low standards of care that are brought about by poverty and ignorance, and those that result from lack of parental care or concern. She concludes that we often cannot, but that nevertheless, children's experiences of serious neglect and its consequences should override, at least initially, concerns about parental culpability and the rights and wrongs of intervention. Stevenson (1998) points to the case of an 18-month-old child named Paul, who died in appalling circumstances as a result of neglect by his parents (Bridge 1995a), as evidence of the fatal consequences that can result from hesitant intervention. Polansky *et al.* (1983) carried out surveys among lay people and found that there were commonly held minimal standards about neglect that could be used to justify child protection investigations.

Despite these findings, the issue of standards of care and the concerns about parental culpability make tackling neglect a very problematic issue for social workers. In addition, the lack of a clear definition makes it problematical to prove neglect in court. The net result is that such cases are less likely to be vigorously pursued than other forms of abuse.[6]

These concerns are particularly pertinent as a result of changes in the 1989 Children Act. Section 31(10) addresses the issue of how to measure, 'significant harm', which is now the sole ground available for the making of a care or supervision order:

> Where the question of whether harm suffered by a child is significant turns on the child's health or development, his health or development shall be compared with that which could reasonably be expected of a similar child.

Lyon (1989: 205) points out that the sorts of comparisons being required are 'invidious, if not well nigh impossible, but do raise incredible spectres of class, cultural, racial, religious and ethnic considerations'. There can be little doubt that establishing neglect on these grounds simply will not work.

To some degree the approach currently being pursued by the Department of Health may reduce some of the difficulties outlined above. By treating neglect less overtly as abuse, but by ensuring that despite this, it is more adequately responded to in terms of family support, the result may be overall a more positive one.

Failure to thrive

It is notable that the 2000 guidelines do not refer specifically to the 'failure to thrive' syndrome which was included in the 1991 guidelines. Much focus has been placed on this serious potentially life-threatening form of abuse for many years. It has been seen as a syndrome which is technically easier to define and prove than general neglect (see Iwaniec *et al.* 1985). Babies have an expected normal level of growth (weight and length), which is based upon their birth weight and size. Those that fall well below this expectation, with no apparent physical explanation, are considered to be causes for concern; neglect (both physical and emotional) is thought to be a likely cause of this. Close monitoring of a child's physical growth when placed away from the parents may often show that, with reasonable care and feeding, normal development will take place, thus proving that some form of neglect lies at the heart of the problem. The Jasmine Beckford inquiry report (Brent 1985) dealt with this issue in some detail. Jasmine was physically abused and also failing to thrive in terms of physical growth and development. Regular medical checks, had they been arranged, may well have pinpointed the latter as a cause for concern.[7] As a result of this case, there is now more awareness of the need to monitor the physical development of all abused children and greater powers to enforce such monitoring have been created in the 1989 Children Act.

Sexual abuse

Sexual abuse is defined in the 2000 guidelines as involving

> forcing or enticing a child or young person to take part in sexual activities, whether or not the child is aware of what is happening. The activities may involve physical contact, including penetrative (e.g. rape or buggery) and non-penetrative acts. They may include non-contact activities, such as involving children in looking at, or in the production of, pornographic material or watching sexual activities or encouraging children to behave in sexually inappropriate ways.
>
> (DoH 2000a: 6)

This is more helpful as a nominal definition than the brief and vague effort produced in the 1991 guidelines: 'Actual or likely sexual exploitation of a child or adolescent. The child may be dependent and/or emotionally immature' (DoH 1991b: 49). It specifies the fact that sexual abuse need not involve physical contact and it provides some specific

examples of such non-contact abuse. However, there are still many
gaps to be filled. For instance, it makes no distinction between intrafamilial and extrafamilial abuse, and it says nothing about the age of
the perpetrator. Glaser and Frosh's (1988) definition still seems to be
more comprehensive than that offered in official guidance:

> Any child below the age of consent may be deemed to have been
> sexually abused when a sexually mature person has, by design or
> by neglect of their usual societal or specific responsibilities in
> relation to the child, engaged or permitted the engagement of
> that child in any activity of a sexual nature which is intended to
> lead to the sexual gratification of the sexually mature person. This
> definition pertains whether or not it involves genital contact or
> physical contact, and whether or not there is discernible harmful
> outcome in the short-term.
>
> (Glaser and Frosh 1988: 5)

The issue of defining sexual abuse in practice is both complex and
problematical. There is now general awareness that child sexual abuse
is not only far more common but also affects much younger children
than was previously considered to be the case (see Macfarlane and
Waterman 1986). Child health and welfare professionals are now largely
agreed that sexual abuse of children is a very serious form of abuse
and that intervention to protect children from such abuse in whatever
form is a very high priority. However, there are major problems in
gathering evidence to prove suspicions. In what follows, it should be
noted that the focus is on intrafamilial abuse. This is largely because
this form of abuse lies more squarely in the domain of social work.
However, the importance of responding to the needs of children and
families where the former have experienced abuse outside the family
should not be underestimated (see Fischer and Macdonald 1998 for
useful information on similarities and differences between these two
forms of sexual abuse).

Medical, social and behavioural factors in defining sexual abuse

There are few clear-cut medical signs of abuse. Thus, most medical
examinations of children suspected of having been abused yield little
by way of evidence. As we saw in Chapter 4, following the Cleveland
inquiry there is now a good deal of circumspection about certain
types of medical evidence that previously were beginning to be considered to be more definite indicators. It is now generally accepted
that medical evidence without some form of corroboration from a
social and behavioural assessment is not sufficient to prove child sexual
abuse in court. However, it is also difficult to be definite about social
and behavioural assessments. It is generally thought that sexual abuse

of children is a cross-class phenomenon (see Finkelhor *et al.* 1986: 66) and is as common among more 'respectable' families as it is in families that normally come under the surveillance of welfare agencies. With regard to behavioural indicators, a variety of factors have been identified as associated with sexual abuse of children, for example precocious sexual behaviour, withdrawn presentation, parasuicide and suicide, running away from home and anorexia nervosa (see Porter 1984). However, these correlations do not prove connections and can, therefore, only sensitize professionals to the possibility of sexual abuse. They have very little value in terms of the standard of evidence required in courts.

The child's testimony

Because of this lack of hard scientific evidence and because of the very secretive nature of intrafamilial sexual abuse of children (Furniss 1991), which makes it unlikely that anyone but the perpetrator and the child know that the abuse is going on, the child's account of events is a crucial factor. It is also, however, a controversial issue. Although there is general acceptance among front-line professional workers that children do not lie about being sexually abused, lawyers, in particular, have pointed to cases and situations in which children can and do make false allegations (see Mantell 1988). The Cleveland report considered that social workers and clinical psychologists were too uncritical in their adherence to belief in the child, and saw this as contributing to their generally over-zealous approach in disclosure interviews (Butler-Sloss 1988: 204–9). A consequence of this has been that social work evidence of child sexual abuse based on such interviews is now treated in court with a good deal of scepticism. The acceptability of a child's evidence in criminal court is another problematic issue affecting proof of sexual abuse. Prior to the implementation of the 1998 Criminal Justice Act, a child's evidence could not be accepted unless it was corroborated by some other evidence, making conviction of alleged offenders far less likely. However, following this and the implementation of the subsequent 1991 Criminal Justice Act, corroboration of such evidence is no longer a compulsory requirement and videos of children alleging abuse can be used as evidence in court, provided that the child is available for cross-examination (see Cobley 1995). Nevertheless, there is still tremendous pressure placed on children in such proceedings (Flin 1990) and this acts as a deterrent to those deciding whether to prosecute alleged offenders or not.

Living with uncertainty

There is, therefore, currently a good deal of uncertainty about decisions in this field because of the great difficulty associated with proving that the abuse has happened. The general effects of Cleveland have been to create a more cautious approach following a period when there was growing confidence about the way ahead. There now seems to be a good deal of suspected child sexual abuse, but more circumspection about defining it as such and acting on that suspicion without more definite proof (see Corby 1998).

Emotional abuse

Emotional abuse for the purposes of registration is defined in the 2000 Department of Health guidelines as

> the persistent emotional ill-treatment of a child such as to cause severe and persistent adverse effects on the child's emotional development. It may involve conveying to the children that they are worthless or unloved, inadequate, or valued only insofar as they meet the needs of another person. It may feature age or developmentally inappropriate expectations being placed on children. It may involve causing children frequently to feel frightened, or the exploitation or corruption of children. Some level of emotional abuse is involved in all types of ill-treatment of a child, though it may occur alone.
>
> (DoH 2000a: 5–6)

Defining emotional abuse for practical intervention purposes is extremely difficult. Social workers seem to be particularly aware of and concerned about the emotional ill-treatment of children, but find it very hard to pinpoint their concerns. This is because they are tackling areas of major uncertainty and sensitivity, which are both controversial and difficult to prove. Styles of parenting are brought into question by the issue of emotional abuse. For instance, are authoritarian or extremely permissive parenting styles abusive? Is constant criticism of a child an abuse? Can it be proved that such parenting styles have ill-effects? Where is the line between acceptable and unacceptable psychological parenting to be drawn? Is it abusive actively to prejudice a child against people of different races and sexes? Some would argue this to be so, but would be hard pressed to prove that such upbringings are actively harmful to those individuals, even though it is likely that society as a whole will be the poorer for such forms of socialization. It is difficult to prove links between causes and effects in this area; Garbarino and Vondra (1987) describe 'stress-resistant' children who despite apparently rejecting parents survive to be reasonably well-adjusted adults.

Given these problems, some, like Goldstein et al. (1979), argue that there should be no intervention into this type of case at all on the grounds that it is likely to have more harmful consequences than non-intervention. Wald (1982) supports limited coercive intervention only where the minor is suffering serious emotional damage, evidenced by severe anxiety, depression or withdrawal, or untoward aggressive behaviour or hostility towards others, and the parents are unwilling to provide treatment for the child.

Garbarino and Gilliam (1980), however, use a broad definition that gives professionals a good deal of discretion. They define what they term psychological maltreatment as 'Acts of omission or commission by a parent or guardian that are judged by a mixture of community values and professional expertise to be inappropriate and damaging' (Garbarino and Gilliam 1980: 7). How such a definition could be operationalized is hard to envisage. Burnett (1993) has tried to develop a more specific set of definitions. Using vignettes with the public and professionals in a moderate sized city in north-east USA, he found general agreement on nine forms of what he termed psychological abuse:

1 confining a child in a small place
2 severe public humiliation
3 the 'Cinderella' syndrome
4 severe verbal abuse
5 encouraging or coercing a child into delinquency
6 threatening a child
7 refusal of psychiatric treatment
8 not allowing social and emotional growth
9 not providing a loving, nurturing atmosphere.

(Burnett 1993: 446)

However, there was still much uncertainty (more among professionals than the public) on how the state could intervene to protect children in these situations. The most common current view on the issue seems to be that emotional abuse and neglect of children is in itself damaging, but for practical purposes it has to have identifiable serious consequences linked to parenting behaviour before it can be statutorily responded to (see Montgomery 1989).

Factors common to all types of abuse

It has to be stressed that there may be overlaps and connections between the different forms of abuse. Thus, a child may be physically and sexually abused, physically abused and neglected and so on. As the 2000 DoH guidelines stress, emotional abuse, while theoretically able to occur by itself, is also almost certain to accompany or be a consequence of the other forms of abuse. Until the late 1980s, the emotional impact of physical abuse and neglect received little attention. This has been less true in the case of sexual abuse because it was largely the harrowing stories of survivors of such abuse that brought the problem to the public's attention. Currently, the emotional or psychological effects of all forms of abuse are being seen as a unifying factor in identifying and responding to them. Focus on the emotional aspects of abuse is seen as a way of moving forward more positively to improving the quality of life of all children who experience any form of mistreatment. As Garbarino and Vondra (1987) put it:

> Rather than casting psychological maltreatment as an ancillary issue (subordinate to other forms of abuse and neglect) we should place it as the centre-piece of our efforts to understand famly functioning and to protect children.
>
> (Garbarino and Vondra 1987: 28)

Other forms of abuse

There are a wide range of other forms of child mistreatment about which concern has been expressed.

Other concerns stemming from paediatrics

We have considered several medically derived concerns found in the child protection guidelines. There are some that have not been mentioned. The first is psychosocial short stature syndrome, formerly termed deprivation dwarfism. This is a syndrome identified by paediatricians whereby growth of children becomes stunted as a result of emotional or physical neglect. It is similar to the failure-to-thrive syndrome, but usually becomes apparent only in older children and can cause physical development to be permanently impaired (Gardner 1972).

Second, there is what is termed 'foetal abuse'. This has been a concern for some time in the USA and there have been cases brought before the British courts. It is a term used in relation to behaviours on the part of a pregnant mother, such as excessive use of tobacco, alcohol and prohibited drugs that are considered harmful to the unborn child (Mackenzie *et al.* 1982).

A third, more recent concern of paediatricians relates to the actual abuse of children detained in hospital by their parents. This has led to a controversial form of intervention using covert video surveillance of parents visiting their children. It has been developed in Staffordshire and entails admitting to hospital wards younger children who have aroused concerns because of poor physical and emotional development, and secretly observing interactions between them and their parents. The paediatricians found high rates of abuse during visits and video tapes have been used to provide evidence in criminal proceedings (Southall *et al.* 1997). While the concerns of the medical profession are to crack the problem of properly ascertaining illness-induced abuse, critics see these practices as a form of entrapment (Thomas 1996).

Institutional, ritual and organized abuse

The background to concerns about these forms of abuse was discussed in Chapter 4. As noted there, these forms of abuse involve both physical and sexual mistreatment. Linked to these forms of abuse are concerns about abuse in foster care (see Utting 1997).

Bullying

The bullying of children by their peers in settings away from home has also been referred to earlier (see Sinclair and Gibbs 1998). Bullying of children in day schools has traditionally been seen as a school behaviour problem falling within the province of education authorities, but more and more linkages are being made between behaviours outside the family and those within. Thus physical bullying, sexual bullying and rape in schools are viewed as possible symptoms of intrafamilial abuse as well as abuses or crimes in their own right.

There are particular concerns about racist bullying which was the subject of concern in the Burnage report (Macdonald 1990) and is currently a high profile issue following the publication of the Stephen Lawrence inquiry report (Macpherson 1999).

Child prostitutes, child runaways and child pornography

There have been considerable developments in official thinking about child prostitution. Up to the mid-1990s, child prostitutes have been seen primarily as young offenders rather than as children in need or as abused children (see Ennew 1986; Jesson 1993). Child-focused work carried out by voluntary agencies like Barnardo's (1998) has been the catalyst for a change of thinking in this respect as have cases of children in care being involved in prostitution. These developments led to the issue of a joint Home Office and Department of Health draft circular in 1998 promoting an approach whereby the children involved in prostitution should primarily be treated as victims of child abuse.

Similar concerns and rethinking are currently being voiced about child runaways, both from their own homes and care (Biehal *et al.* 1995). There are concerns about rising numbers and greater sensitivity to the fact that running away may be caused by abuse in the settings from which they have absconded.

Child pornography is yet another concern which is currently prominent. The 1999 guidelines specifically refer to child pornography on the Internet. They advise the following:

As part of their role in preventing abuse and neglect, ACPCs [Area Child Protection Committees] may wish to consider activities to raise awareness about the safe use of the Internet by children, for example, by distributing information through education staff to parents, in relation to both school and home-based use of computers by children.

(DoH 2000a: 73)

Domestic violence and mental health

Returning to the family, there has been much greater awareness of links between abuse of women by their partners and physical abuse (see Farmer and Owen 1995). Also, as referred to earlier, there is much greater sensitivity to the impact of this form of violence on children's emotional development (see Henning et al. 1997).

Research by Falkov (1996) into the deaths of children who have been the subject of Part 8 Reviews shows a relatively high number of mental health problems particularly with mothers. Although this is not necessarily a cause of abuse, nor is it a form of abuse, it is important to include this form of concern in a review of issues relating to definitions.

Concluding comments

As can be seen, what is defined as child abuse has grown and grown from the battered child of 1962 to a vast range of practices and behaviours. The field is a very complex one: increasingly welfare professionals are being required to take on new issues and concerns, even though their primary focus will continue to be on the main forms of intrafamilial abuse – physical, sexual, emotional and neglect.

However, it is also clear that despite this broadening of concerns, paradoxically the focus is still quite a narrow one compared with the range of concerns that exist about children internationally, such as child labour, children living in war zones and children of the streets. Harris (1995) has pointed out how culturally specific and selective our concerns are in relation to identifying and defining child abuse.

This is undoubtedly true and consideration of the international scene should provide some perspective on domestic concerns without reducing any commitment to tackling them. Awareness of these matters and the complexities involved in defining child abuse in our own society which have been thus far reviewed should sensitize professionals to the changing and subjective nature of assessing child abuse concerns and to the need to develop clear thinking and objective criteria for this purpose.

Recommended reading

Besharov, D. (1981) Towards better research on child abuse and neglect: making definitional issues an explicit methodological concern, *Child Abuse and Neglect*, 5: 383–90.

Department of Health (1995) *Child Protection: Messages from Research*. London: HMSO.

Giovannoni, J. and Becerra, R. (1979) *Defining Child Abuse*. New York: Free Press.

Gough, D. (1996) Defining the problem, *Child Abuse and Neglect*, 20: 993–1002.

Stevenson, O. (1998) *Neglected Children: Issues and Dilemmas*. Oxford: Blackwell.

chapter **six**

THE EXTENT OF CHILD ABUSE

While it may not be of direct relevance to day-to-day decision-making in the fieldwork office or the clinic to know how widespread child abuse is, such information does have an influence on the policy-maker who determines resource allocation and the structures for responding to child abuse situations and, therefore, indirectly on practice. In addition, knowledge gained from incidence and prevalence studies and from official statistics can to some extent contextualize child protection work by giving a sense of the whole. It can also, as we shall see, pose important questions about the effects of past and present policies and practice and point to ways forward.

There are two main sources of statistical knowledge. The first, drawn largely from government departments, measures the incidence of child abuse as reported, recorded or registered by official agencies. The second, deriving from a broader research base, measures the incidence and prevalence of abuse in a given sample of people.[1] Thus, official statistics tell us more about the way in which child abuse is defined in practice and responded to over time, whereas research studies tell us more about the 'hidden' problem, that is abuse that does not come to the attention of those officially authorized to deal with it.

Official statistics

Any figures relating to child protection work need to be carefully analysed because of the definitional complications considered in Chapter 5. There are four sets of official statistics that will be referred to here:

- child protection statistics in Britain
- child protection statistics in the USA
- numbers of children in care
- childhood mortality statistics.

Child protection statistics in Britain

Until 1988, there were no national statistics kept in Britain with regard to the officially known extent of child abuse. To obtain a national picture before this, use was made of the returns of the NSPCC special unit registers, which covered approximately 9 per cent of the child population of England and Wales. From 1988, figures have been available from the Department of Health, which now annually collates the numbers of children on child protection registers in England. While there are many problems associated with interpretation of these statistics because of variations in practice between local authorities (see Corby 1990), they nevertheless provide at least some tools with which to assess and monitor trends of practice in general terms.

Table 6.1 Total numbers of children on child protection registers in England and Wales for selected years between 1978 and 1999

Year	Number on register	Source
1978	11,844	Creighton (1984)
1984	12,389	Creighton (1985)
1985	17,622	Creighton (1986)
1986	23,820	Creighton (1987)
1987	29,766	Association of the Directors of Social Services (1988)
1988	39,200 (England only)	DoH (1989)
1989	41,200 (England only)	DoH (1990)
1990	43,600 (England only)	DoH (1991c)
1991	45,200 (England only)	DoH (1992)
1992	38,600 (England only)	DoH (1993)
1995	35,000 (England only)	DoH (1996)
1999	31,900 (England only)	DoH (1999c)

Table 6.1 has been devised using extrapolations from the NSPCC figures and those from the Department of Health. These figures show nearly a fourfold increase in numbers of children on child protection registers between 1984 and 1991. Whereas in 1984 one in every thousand children was registered, the rate in 1991 was four per thousand.

This rise in numbers of children registered was a clear reflection of the growth of child protection concerns and the increased formalization of child protection processes.

The 1990s saw a gradual decline in the number of children on registers – the rate was just under three per thousand in 1999. As can be seen there was a sharp decline in numbers on the register between 1991 and 1992. This followed on from the elimination of the grave concern category as a result of which there was need for more specificity about the causes of concern before registration could be completed. Another factor which accounts for the decline is increased throughput of cases with greater use of deregistration. As can be seen from Table 6.2, there was a 65 per cent increase in the number of deregistrations between 1988 and 1999.

It should be noted that the annual rate of registration has also increased between these years by approximately one-third. Thus the impression of a decline in child protection concerns in the 1990s given by Table 6.1 is not borne out by the figures in Table 6.2. In terms of actual activity (as opposed to absolute numbers) child protection work has been on the increase since 1990.

A breakdown of the numbers of children on registers according to different categories of abuse (Table 6.3) provides more detail about the

Table 6.2 Registrations to and deregistrations from child protection registers for selected years ending 31 March 1988–1999

Year	Registrations	Deregistrations
1988	20,900	17,900
1991	28,300	26,700
1995	30,400	30,200
1999	30,100	29,600

Table 6.3 Numbers of children on child protection registers in England and Wales by category for selected years between 1978 and 1999

Category of abuse	1978	1984	1986	1988	1991	1995	1999
Physical abuse	7,944	7,856	10,422	11,100	9,000	12,300	6,500
Physical neglect	289	933	1,888	4,900	5,600	9,200	11,100
Sexual abuse	89	1,088	5,922	5,800	5,600	7,200	4,800
Emotional abuse	0	200	455	1,700	2,600	3,800	5,400
Grave concern	3,522	2,312	5,133	14,400	21,100	—	—
Total	11,844	12,389	23,820	39,200	45,200	35,000	31,900

Note: Totals for 1988, 1991, 1995 and 1999 include small numbers of children registered under joint categories. Figures for 1988–99 are for England only. Sources are as for Table 6.1.

nature of the development of official child protection work in Britain over the same period.

The proportion of children registered on account of being physically abused has fallen considerably. Whereas in 1978 the physical abuse category accounted for 67 per cent of the total children registered, by 1999 the proportion had fallen to below one-third. In 1978, neglect cases constituted just under 5 per cent of the whole. By 1999, neglect cases constituted 42 per cent of the total numbers on registers, the largest of the categories, and this is despite more emphasis on working in a more family supportive way with cases where serious abuse has not been assessed.

Child sexual abuse cases were a very minor concern of the authorities in 1978, forming less than 1 per cent of the whole. In 1991, they formed just over 11 per cent of the total. By 1999 sexual abuse cases constituted 19 per cent of the total having declined gradually from a high of 24 per cent in 1995.

Emotional abuse of children did not officially exist in 1978. By 1999, emotionally abused children made up 16 per cent of the total number registered.

The grave concern category formed nearly 30 per cent of the whole in 1978 and just under 50 per cent of the whole in 1991. It was something of a miscellaneous category, originally incorporating cases where those convicted of offences against children had been living or were about to live in the same household as children, and cases where there had been strong suspicions of physical abuse, sexual abuse or neglect, but no definite evidence. As pointed out earlier, this category was abandoned at the end of 1991. It is likely that the increase in neglect and emotional abuse cases between 1991 and 1999 is partly as a result of the elimination of this category.

The pattern of events is relatively clear. Between 1978 and 1991, the focus of child abuse concerns shifted from almost exclusive emphasis on the physical abuse of children to a broader range of forms of child maltreatment. This broader focus was maintained throughout the 1990s during which time the amount of child protection activity judged by registrations and deregistrations remained fairly constant. The greatest rise was among cases of physical and emotional neglect. Given the wide range of new child protection concerns considered in Chapter 5, such as institutionalized abuse and child prostitution, it might be asked whether the categories should be made more specific.

These figures have largely dealt with cases at the end of the process. Research by Gibbons et al. (1995a) also provides some useful statistics about how the child protection system deals with the total number of referrals it receives. Gibbons and her colleagues examined all child protection referrals made to eight local authority social services departments over a six-month period. Extrapolating from this research, it is estimated over a year that:

- 160,000 referrals about child protection concerns are made
- 120,000 of these referrals result in family visits
- 40,000 of these result in child protection conferences
- 11,000 of these result in no further action
- 24,500 registrations take place
- 3000 children are worked with on a voluntary basis
- 6000 children come into the care of the local authority as a result (3000 through care proceedings).

Child protection statistics in the USA

The pattern of events demonstrated by the British statistics is similar to that which has taken place in the USA; the main difference is that it took place earlier there. In 1968, according to Gil (1970), there were 10,931 reports of child abuse in the USA, of which 6617 were confirmed cases, that is 1 in every 10,000 children under the age of 18. The bulk of these cases were of physical abuse. A national incidence study estimated that there were 1,151,600 suspected child abuse cases in 1979–80, of which 652,000 were substantiated (100 per 10,000 children). Just under 33 per cent of these cases were concerned with physical abuse, 7 per cent were cases of sexual abuse and about 60 per cent were cases of physical and emotional neglect (National Center on Child Abuse and Neglect 1981). By 1986, the number of suspected cases had risen to 1.6 million (National Center on Child Abuse and Neglect 1986). In 1997 (see Elders 1999) there were 3,195,000 reports of child abuse made to child protection agencies, of which approximately 1 million were substantiated on follow-up (150 per 10,000 children). Of these cases 52 per cent came under the category of neglect, 24 per cent were physical abuse and 24 per cent were made up of sexual and emotional abuse cases.

Thus the same sort of expansion has taken place in the USA as in Britain, but on a far greater scale. Assuming substantiated cases in the USA to be the equivalent of children on child protection registers in Britain, the American system now identifies as at risk five times more children than in Britain. There is some reason to believe that the American system incorporates more moderate cases than does the British system. However, even allowing for this, the gap between the rates of intervention is considerable. Nevertheless, as we have seen, the debate in Britain centres around reducing the number of children being formally investigated for child protection reasons on the assumption that our systems are over-interventional.

Numbers of children in care

Children in care statistics published annually by the Department of Health give further information about the way in which child protection cases are responded to. The total numbers of children in care/looked after declined consistently between 1987 and 1994 from approximately 65,000 to 49,300. However, since 1994 the numbers have gradually risen again, reaching 55,300 in 1999. The statistics do not enable us to calculate the absolute numbers of children in care at any one time as a result of child abuse. However, the percentage of children in care as a result of care proceedings has increased overall between 1984 and 1999 which might be interpreted as evidence of an increase in numbers of abused or neglected children in care.

Somewhat paradoxically, the number of children starting to be looked after in any one year decreased slightly in the 1994–9 period. Thus the rise in the numbers actually in care is a result of children being looked after longer. There are statistics that do show the number of children coming into care in any one year as a result of child abuse or neglect. In 1997, 23 per cent of the intake came into care for that reason (7200). This compares with 14 per cent in 1993 (4200). Thus, despite the decline in the numbers of children starting to be looked after between 1994 and 1999, more of these children have been abused or neglected. Also more have started to be looked after as a result of care proceedings and slightly more children in care are on child protection registers (7900 in 1999 compared with 7600 in 1994). These figures are somewhat surprising given the fact that they seem to run contrary to the direction favoured by public policy during this period.

Overall, the figures suggest that except in the case of short-term admissions, children who have been abused or neglected are increasingly dominating the children in care scene.

Child mortality statistics

Another source of information about the extent of child abuse is to be found in child mortality statistics. These statistics are collated by the Office of Population and Census Statistics. There are two sets – those relating to the deaths of children aged from birth to 14 years of age from homicide and those caused by undetermined injuries whether accidentally or purposely inflicted. Table 6.4 shows the general trends between 1973 and 1992.

Table 6.4   Deaths of children aged 0–14 from homicide and undetermined injuries, 1973–92

Years	Total child homicides	Total child undetermined deaths	Total deaths
1973–82	770	488	1258
1983–92	442	579	1021
Ratio of change	0.57	1.2	0.81

Source: Pritchard 1996: 551

These figures show a considerable decrease in the number of deaths from homicide between 1973 and 1992. In 1973 there were 102 child deaths by homicide, and in 1992 there were 29. However, there has been an increase in the number of child deaths through injuries where the causes were undetermined. The comparative figures for 1973 and 1992 were 56 and 81 respectively. Taking both sets of figures, however, there has been a 20 per cent decrease in the number of child deaths in the 1983–92 decade compared with the preceding decade.

Pritchard (1992, 1996) has drawn attention to these statistics and used them to argue that both in themselves, and in comparison with statistics from other European countries, they are indicators of the success of the child protection system that was developed in Britain following the Maria Colwell inquiry report. His claim, however, has been subjected to much criticism. Creighton (1993) argued that there was a change in recording child deaths in 1979 that led to a sharp reduction in the number of child homicides, and an increase in the number of deaths by undetermined injuries. Lindsey and Trocme (1994) raised several telling points. First, they argued that the base rates of child homicide are so low that great care needs to be made in using them to assume trends. Second, they pointed to the fact that many deaths by homicide and undetermined injuries are not classical child abuse deaths; they include single assault deaths, murders followed by the suicide of a parent or parents and murders by strangers (particularly in the case of adolescents). Given that child deaths include such a wide range of circumstances, many of which are not the types of cases in which social workers are likely to be involved, it is, therefore, considered to be fallacious to attribute declining death rates to the success of the child protection system. Macdonald (1995) also questioned whether child deaths are a useful indicator of effectiveness of intervention, given that most child protection work is done with families where there is little risk of fatalities.

Incidence and prevalence studies into child abuse

Incidence and prevalence studies are survey based. Researchers seek by interview and questionnaire to find out how many children in a general population are subjected to maltreatment and how often (see note 1). Definitional issues are very important in the assessment of the value of different studies. So too are methodological concerns, such as the representativeness of the sample and the way in which the research is conducted, for example by direct questioning, mailed questionnaire or telephone interview.

Consideration will be given to studies into the incidence and prevalence of physical abuse and neglect first and then sexual abuse. One very obvious difference between the research methodologies in these two areas is the fact that, in the case of physical abuse, generally parents are asked about their use of physical violence against their children, whereas, with regard to sexual abuse, the survivor, not the perpetrator, is the provider of the information. One obvious consequence of this is the expectation that the former will provide a conservative estimate of the true extent of physical abuse.

Physical abuse studies

In Britain

There have been no large-scale studies into the incidence and prevalence of physical abuse in Britain. There have, however, been several studies looking at the use of physical punishment by parents, which (as we saw in Chapter 5) is coming more and more to be seen by many concerned with child protection issues as having some linkages with more serious child abuse. Leach (1999) has produced a useful summary of recent research referring particularly to data by Newson and Newson (1989) and Nobes and Smith (1997). In a longitudinal study of 700 families in Nottingham, Newson and Newson (1989) found that two-thirds of parents had smacked their babies by the time of their first birthdays. By age 4, more than nine out of ten children were smacked at least weekly. By the time children were 7, almost one-quarter of parents were regularly hitting their children with straps and sticks and other implements. Nobes and Smith (1997) came to similar findings. They noted in addition that children with two resident parents usually received twice the punishment of a child with a lone parent, that women tended to underestimate the punitiveness of their male partners and that 35 per cent of children aged 11 had been subjected at some time to 'severe' punishment.

In the USA

More extensive work into the issue of abusive violence towards children has been conducted in the USA. The most influential research was conducted by Straus and his colleagues. They completed large-scale studies in 1975 and 1985 and compared the results. The first study was based on face-to-face interviews with 1146 parents with a referent child between the ages of 3 and 17.[2] They were asked whether they had been physically violent towards this child on at least one occasion in the past 12 months. This study was repeated in 1985 with 1428 parents in similar circumstances. This second study was conducted by telephone interview. The results are set out in Table 6.5.

Straus and Gelles (1986) argued that these studies demonstrate that, between 1975 and 1985, general violence to children has stayed at about the same level. However, the prevalence of severe violence has declined by 24 per cent and that of very severe violence, which the researchers equated with child abuse, by 47 per cent. They attributed this change to a variety of social and economic factors, including the development of child protection strategies and programmes. Stocks (1988) questioned the validity of these conclusions, largely on methodological grounds.

An adequate response?

Regardless of the issue of the effectiveness of child protection systems, the studies do demonstrate that the annual prevalence of severe and very severe physical child abuse (that is 126 per 1000), as measured by

Table 6.5 Comparison of parent-to-child violence in 1975 and 1985

	Rate per 1000 children aged 3–17	
Type of violence	1975	1985
Minor violence acts		
1 Threw something	54	27
2 Pushed, grabbed, shoved	318	307
3 Slapped or spanked	582	549
Severe violence acts		
4 Kicked, bit, hit with fist	32	13
5 Hit, tried to hit with something	134	97
6 Beat up	13	6
7 Threatened with gun or knife	1	2
8 Used gun or knife	1	2
Violence indexes		
Overall violence (1–8)	630	620
Severe violence (4–8)	140	107
Very severe violence (4, 6, 8)	36	19

Source: Straus and Gelles 1986: 469

direct questioning of parents, which (as we have already noted) is likely to be a conservative estimate, far outstrips the rate of official detection in Britain and to a lesser extent that of the USA. Thus, despite the considerable growth of the child protection machinery, there are far more maltreated children going unnoticed than being protected. Studies of this kind pose particularly important questions for policy-makers, such as whether there is the political will to eliminate all child abuse. If there is, then considerably more resources will be required to achieve that goal than are currently available. Incidence and prevalence studies demonstrate the enormity of the problem to be tackled.

It should be noted that there are other studies of physical child abuse prevalence. Birchall (1989) listed 19 British and US studies between 1952 and 1986. However, many of these are extrapolations from small samples and many are also now somewhat dated.

Considering the publicity that physical abuse of children has received since the early 1970s, it is surprising that there has been so little detailed research into its general incidence in Britain. Currently we are having to guess the total size of the problem and are reliant on data from another country to give us a rough idea. There can be little doubt, therefore, that there is a particular need for much more information on this topic. It should also be noted that we have no detailed information on the extent of neglect or emotional abuse in Britain or the USA which to some extent is linked to the definitional difficulties outlined in Chapter 5.

Sexual abuse prevalence studies

Studies of the prevalence of sexual abuse have been abundant since the early 1980s. Again research into this field has been more evident in the USA than in Britain, but there are more British studies in existence than in the case of physical abuse. Having said this, however, the US studies are generally more sophisticated methodologically and broader in scope. These will therefore be considered first.

In the USA

The results of these studies are very wide-ranging and at first sight somewhat confusing. Finkelhor (1994) found 19 studies conducted in the USA and Canada since 1980. The rates of sexual abuse in these studies varied from 6 to 62 per cent for females and 3 to 16 per cent for males. Finkelhor indicated that prevalence rates of 20 per cent for women and between 5 and 10 per cent for men were reasonable summary statistics. He attributed this wide variation in rates to several factors. These included:

- The lack of standard definitions of child sexual abuse. (Some studies adopt broad definitions, others use narrow definitions. For instance, some studies incorporate non-contact sexual abuse in their definition, others do not. Some studies include extrafamilial abuse in their definitions whereas others do not.)
- The lack of a standard upper age limit. (Some studies adopt an upper age limit of 15, others 18.)
- The lack of agreement about the age difference between the abused child and the perpetrator. (Some studies do not consider this a factor at all. Others use five and ten year age gaps as defining factors.)
- Different sample selections. (Some studies are drawn from college students only, while others are drawn from a more diverse background in terms of class and age.)
- Different forms of data collection. (Some studies use face-to-face interviews with trained interviewers, which seem to elicit higher incidences than do more impersonal approaches.)

Finkelhor's (1979) own survey study in the late 1970s was of 796 college students. It was a questionnaire study, included non-contact and extrafamilial abuse, set the upper age limit for abuse at 16 and specified age gaps between abusers and perpetrators. He found that

19 per cent of women and 9 per cent of men had experienced some kind of sexual abuse during childhood.

Russell (1984) surveyed a community sample of 930 women in San Francisco. In total, 647 incidents of child sexual abuse were disclosed to her interviewers. The definitions she used were as follows:

> Extrafamilial child sexual abuse: one or more unwanted sexual experiences with persons unrelated by blood or marriage, ranging from attempted petting (touching of breasts or genitals, or attempts at such touching) to rape, before the victim turned 14 years, and attempted forcible rape experiences from the ages of 14 to 17 years inclusive.

> Incestuous child abuse: any kind of exploitive sexual contact or attempted sexual contact, that occurred between relatives, no matter how distant the relationship, before the victim turned 18 years old.
>
> (Russell 1984: 180–1)

Russell found that 152 women (16 per cent of the 930 women sampled) reported at least one experience of incestuous abuse before the age of 18 years. Of these, 108 had been sexually abused before the age of 14. Russell also found that 290 women (31 per cent) had experienced extrafamilial abuse before the age of 18 (and 189 before the age of 14). In all, these 290 abused women had 461 experiences of being abused. These results are seen to be at the high end of the spectrum. Russell's interviewers (all female) certainly probed further and more persistently than was the case in other studies. However, Russell (1984) pointed out that many cases of non-contact abuse were recounted, which were not included in the figures. The inclusion of these incidents raised the overall rate of abuse to 54 per cent. Russell also rated the seriousness of the incestuous child abuse incidents. She found that 23 per cent of the cases were very serious (genital–genital and oral–genital contact), 40 per cent serious and 36 per cent less serious. The ratios for extrafamilial abuse were 53 per cent very serious, 27 per cent serious and 20 per cent less serious.

Finkelhor et al. (1990) reported on a national survey carried out in 1985. A total of 1481 women and 1145 men were interviewed by telephone. The definitions used included contact and non-contact abuse by any person. The survey found that 27 per cent of the women and 16 per cent of the men had a history of sexual abuse; 19 per cent of the female victims and 62 per cent of the male victims had experienced actual or attempted sexual intercourse; 29 per cent of the girl victims were abused by family members compared with 11 per cent of the boys; the boys were more likely to be abused by strangers (40 per cent compared with 21 per cent for girls).

It is hard to generalize about these studies. However, one fact that they all emphasize is that child sexual abuse is far more prevalent than would have been considered possible in the early 1980s. Most commentators argue that studies are likely to produce an underestimate of the real incidence of sexual abuse of children because of the shame attached to it and the fact that survivors are likely to have repressed the memory of it. A second commonly emphasized finding is that girls are more vulnerable than boys. Finkelhor *et al.* (1986) in a study of studies carried out in the mid-1980s found that the overall ratio was 79:21, but felt that for various social reasons men were less likely to disclose incidents of sexual abuse than women and, therefore, that the true ratios were closer than this figure suggests. Russell's (1984) study showed that over half of all women are subjected to some form of sexual abuse before the age of 18. Clearly social work intervention would be inappropriate in all such cases. Nevertheless, figures of 16 per cent of all women experiencing some form of incestuous abuse, two-thirds of which is deemed very serious or serious, is a sobering thought for both young females and agencies mandated to provide them with some protection. The later Finkelhor study (Finkelhor *et al.* 1990) pointed to 10 per cent intrafamilial abuse which, given the lower rate of abuse of boys (who in contrast to girls are just as likely to be abused by strangers as in the home), lends support to the rate found by Russell (1984).

In Britain

Mrazek *et al.* (1983) surveyed medical professions to get an estimate of the prevalence of child sexual abuse. They found a rate of 0.3 per cent, which is generally accepted as being a vast underestimate of the total size of the problem. Nash and West (1985) carried out a study of 315 young women and students in Cambridge and found that 48 per cent had experienced some form of abuse. Approximately 25 per cent reported non-contact abuse and 82 per cent were abused in the first instance by non-family abusers. Thus, there is evidence in this study that half of all women are subjected to some form of sexual abuse as children, but it is largely of a kind that may not require the sort of intrafamilial intervention traditionally carried out by social work agencies. A similar type of study was carried out by Kelly *et al.* (1991) in colleges of further education. Using a very broad definition, they found that 59 per cent of women and 27 per cent of men reported at least one experience of sexual abuse.

The influential MORI Poll survey referred to in Chapter 3 (Baker and Duncan 1985) took a representative sample of 2019 people of all ages over 15 and using the following definition of child sexual abuse asked them if they had ever had such an experience before the age of 16:

A child (i.e. under sixteen) is sexually abused when another person, who is sexually mature, involves the child in other activities which the other person expects to lead to their sexual arousal. This might involve intercourse, touching, exposure of the sexual organs, showing pornographic material or talking about sexual things in an erotic way.

(Baker and Duncan 1985: 458)

Of those questioned, 105 said that they had been sexually abused (12 per cent of women and 8 per cent of men); 14 per cent of those who said that they had been abused said that they had been sexually abused within their own families (1.3 per cent of the whole sample); 51 per cent (4.8 per cent of the whole sample) said that they had been abused by strangers and 35 per cent by someone they knew who was not a relation. Just over half of those abused said that the abuse they had experienced involved no physical contact. Nine people (0.45 per cent of the sample) said they had been subjected to incest involving sexual intercourse with a relative.

These findings are more conservative than those of the US studies. La Fontaine's (1988) review of studies in Britain and the USA comes to the conclusion that the best estimate of the overall extrafamilial and intrafamilial prevalence rate of abuse is 10 per cent and this refers to contact abuse only.

The international picture

Countries other than Britain and the USA have also been concerned to seek out the extent of sexual abuse. Finkelhor (1994) reported on large-scale surveys in 21 countries (largely European, North and Central American, and Australasian). He noted that even more care has to be taken in comparing studies cross-nationally than in one country, because of the wider variations of values, customs, definitions and methodologies. Nevertheless, he reported that all the studies revealed sexual abuse histories in at least 7 per cent of the females and at least 3 per cent of the males, ranging up to 36 per cent of women (in Australia) and 29 per cent of men (South Africa). Finkelhor (1994) concluded:

Studies from a variety of countries suggest that sexual abuse is indeed an international problem. In every locale where it has been sought, researchers have demonstrated its existence at levels high enough to be detected through surveys of a few hundred adults in the general population. These rates are far higher than anything suggested by the level of reported cases in these countries. As such epidemiological studies are available for more and more countries, the responsibility of proof shifts to anyone who would argue that sexual abuse is rare or nonexistent in their locale.

(Finkelhor 1994: 412)

These views are echoed by La Fontaine (1990):

There has been enough research to show that the sexual abuse of children is not a negligible issue or a question of public hysteria but a serious social problem. Even the lowest estimate of its prevalence indicates a large number of children are involved.

(La Fontaine 1990: 68)

This is undeniably true. Returning to the British scene, the prevalence rate of intrafamilial abuse pointed to by the MORI Poll survey is 13 per 1000 and the rate of incest is 4 per 1000. Currently the number of children on child protection registers as a result of sexual abuse is 0.5 per 1000. Thus there is still a lot of work for child protection agencies to do.

Concluding comments

Prevalence and incidence studies of child abuse, while riddled with methodological and definitional problems, can, if carefully interpreted, add to our understanding of the problem. It is important to disentangle from them what is valid and relevant to the concerns of different sectors in society. For instance, Straus and Gelles in their 1975 study (see Gelles and Cornell 1985) found that 75 per cent of children in their sample had been subjected to physical violence at least once in the previous 12 months. Clearly, not all these cases are the concern of child protection agencies, because (as we have seen) violence to children (within limits) is not yet culturally disapproved of in North American and British societies. Child protection agencies are mandated to deal with cases considered to be beyond the norm. However, society as a whole may wish to tackle the broader issue of child correction and child care by developing primary prevention programmes that aim to discourage the use of physical punishment of children. For these purposes, the findings of the Straus and Gelles study are important. Child protection agencies, however, will be more concerned with the amount of abusive violence found in studies, knowledge of which will enable them to seek and deploy appropriate resources.

The position is similar with regard to child sexual abuse. Children are clearly subjected to far more sexual abuse than was previously imagined possible. Nevertheless, not all the abuse is relevant to the particular concerns of child protection agencies. The findings, especially those of the American studies, point to the need for a major cultural change regarding sexual behaviour. Child protection agencies, unless they are much better resourced and given a broader remit, will inevitably continue to focus on intrafamilial abuse. Even so, prevalence studies point to the need for a major rethink about the size of this aspect of the problem and the associated resource implications.

Recommended reading

Birchall, E. (1989) The frequency of child abuse: what do we really know?, in O. Stevenson (ed.) *Child Abuse: Public Policy and Professional Practice*. Hemel Hempstead: Harvester-Wheatsheaf.

Corby, B. (1990) Making use of child protection statistics, *Children and Society*, 4: 304–14.

Department of Health (various years) *Survey of Children and Young Persons on Child Protection Registers*. London: HMSO.

Finkelhor, D. (1994) The international epidemiology of child sexual abuse, *Child Abuse and Neglect*, 18: 409–17.

Lindsey, D. and Trocme, N. (1994) Have child protection efforts reduced child homicides? An examination of the data from Britain and North America, *British Journal of Social Work*, 24: 715–32.

chapter **seven**

WHO ABUSES WHOM

There has been a vast quantity of research, largely in the USA, conducted into the questions of who is most likely to abuse children, and which children are most likely to be on the receiving end of that abuse. The goal of this research has largely been prediction and, therefore, prevention.

First, with regard to the 'who abuses' question, the thinking is that if it is possible to identify those parents (and others) who are most likely to abuse or continue to be dangerous to children, then early and decisive intervention is likely to afford those children greater protection. Second, with regard to the question of who is most likely to be at the receiving end of abuse, it is clear that there is a close association between this and the question of who abuses. Children in close proximity to those with a likelihood of abusing are obviously those who are most at risk. However, not all children in this situation seem to be equally at risk. Some children seem to be singled out for mistreatment and researchers have looked into this aspect of child abuse in some detail.

There is a third related issue, that of why child abuse happens. The question of causation is very closely linked to the question of who abuses and who is abused. Indeed, the interrelationship of these three aspects of the problem of child abuse cannot be sufficiently emphasized. However, for the purposes of analysis, these issues will be looked at separately. In this chapter answers to the questions of who abuses and who is abused will be considered. Theories of causation will be the subject of Chapter 8.

Who abuses

Researchers into the issue of who abuses children have looked at a wide range of variables that they have felt likely to be associated with abusive behaviour. Inevitably, given the amount of research that has been carried out, this summary will be a selective one. The factors selected for closer inspection are as follows:

- the gender of those who abuse
- the age of those who abuse
- poverty, race and child abuse
- parents who have been abused themselves
- family structure and child abuse
- the psychological capacities of those who abuse
- other factors associated with those who abuse children including the impact of alcohol and drugs; social isolation; partner problems and wife abuse; criminality; and pregnancy, prematurity, bonding and other neonatal problems.

The gender of those who abuse

It is generally thought that mothers are mainly responsible for mistreating children in cases of neglect and physical abuse, especially those at the younger end of the spectrum, and that fathers, or father substitutes, are responsible for nearly all acts of intrafamilial sexual abuse of children. Common assumptions about parenting roles and the nature of sexuality probably account for both these views. First, child care is seen to be the responsibility of women and, therefore, when things go wrong the fault is thought to lie with them. This is seen to hold true even in cases where it has been established that a male has been the perpetrator of physical abuse.[1] Second, women's sexual nature is seen to be such that they are thought highly unlikely to abuse children sexually. It is notable that, despite this view, women are still held to be partly responsible for what happens – hence the term 'collusive mothers'.[2]

Physical abuse and neglect

With regard to physical abuse and neglect, research findings are not as helpful as they might be. Many researchers make the assumption that women are the key figures with regard to these forms of abuse. Often they do not clarify who has abused or neglected the child when there are both male and female carers living in the family. In lone-parent families (see pp. 113–14), it is usually assumed that abuse is the responsibility of the lone carer, unless there is evidence to the contrary. In both these situations, there is a likelihood that women might well be over-represented in the abuser category because of beliefs about their roles, responsibilities and natures. In this way researchers replicate the views and practices of social workers and other professionals, who carry out much of their work in such cases almost exclusively with women (see O'Hagan and Dillenberger 1995).

Creighton and Noyes (1989) analysed data on the perpetrators of all forms of abuse reported to the NSPCC between 1983 and 1987. They found that natural mothers were only slightly more frequently implicated as abusers than fathers in cases of physical abuse, much more frequently implicated as abusers in neglect and emotional abuse cases, and considered to play a negligible part in sexual abuse. However, with regard to physical abuse they point out that 'If the data is analysed by who the child was living with at the time then natural mothers were implicated in 36 per cent and natural fathers in 61 per cent of the injury cases where the child was living with them' (Creighton and Noyes 1989: 21). This suggests that children in two-parent families are more likely to be physically abused by their fathers than by their mothers. In addition there is some support for the view that men living with children are more likely than women to abuse them seriously. Creighton (1984), using register returns for 1977–82, found that mothers were implicated in 41.4 per cent of serious injuries to children and fathers in 32.9 per cent, but where there were two parents living together fathers were implicated in 49.1 per cent of cases and mothers in 36.1 per cent. Brewster *et al.* (1998) analysed 32 cases of infanticide on United States Air Force bases between 1989 and 1995. Infanticide is generally thought to be perpetrated by mothers. In this study, however, 84 per cent of the abusers were males looking after children on their own at the time of the fatal abuse episodes. It is also worth noting that many of the child deaths inquired into in Britain are known to be the result of father/male carer abuse, for example Darryn Clarke (DHSS 1979), Jasmine Beckford (Brent 1985), Tyra Henry (Lambeth 1987), Kimberley Carlile (Greenwich 1987) and Sukina (Bridge 1991).

Thus it can be concluded that for a variety of reasons, associated largely with male gender-biased assumptions, women are thought to be more implicated in the physical abuse and neglect of children than is in fact the case.[3]

Sexual abuse

The evidence about the gender of child sexual abuse perpetrators is somewhat more clear-cut. Finkelhor (1984) estimated that 95 per cent of girls and 80 per cent of boys are sexually abused by males. Of 114 women who reported that they had been sexually abused in Nash and West's (1985) study, only one had been abused by a woman. Of 411 sexually abused children referred to the Great Ormond Street Hospital for Sick Children between 1980 and 1986, 8 children (2 per cent) had been abused by females (Ben-Tovim *et al.* 1988).

There are few well-documented profiles of male intrafamilial sex abusers, because much of the material about perpetrators is derived from work carried out with extrafamilial abusers. It may, however, be important to distinguish between the two. Becker and Quinsey (1993: 170) pointed out that 'extrafamilial child molesters are more likely to recidivate than strictly intrafamilial child molesters and men who choose boy victims are more likely to recidivate than men who abuse girl victims'.

There are a small number of studies of intrafamilial female sex abusers. Krug (1989) studied eight cases in detail and came to the conclusion that female sexual abuse of children mirrored that of male sexual abuse:

> The sexual abuse typically involved the mother satisfying her own emotional and physical needs for intimacy, security and perhaps power by actively seeking out the son, either on a nightly basis, or when she and her living [live-in] partner were in conflict.
>
> (Krug 1989: 112)

Others, however, have argued that mother–son abuse is different from abuse by male perpetrators in that it is often less coercive (Lawson 1993).

Banning (1989) considered sexual abuse by females to be on the increase and attributed this development to the blurring of roles between men and women. However, there is a need for some degree of perspective when considering these accounts. While it is wrong to assume that women do not sexually abuse children, one should not fall into the trap of seeing such abuse as perpetrated equally by men and women. As Finkelhor (1984: 184) pointed out, 'to take the appearance of some forms of sexual abuse by women to mean that sexual abuse is not primarily committed by men is also wrong and has no support in any of the data'.

The age of those who abuse

Physical abuse

Traditionally, physical abuse and neglect of children has been associated with young and immature parents. Baldwin and Oliver (1975) and Greenland (1987), in their studies of serious and fatal child abuse cases, both confirmed such an association. Smith et al. (1974: 576) asserted that 'Child abuse is associated with both illegitimacy and prematurity of parenthood'. In their study 54 per cent of mothers had had their first child before the age of 20. Lynch (1975) found the same in 40 per cent of her sample. Hyman (1978) found that the mean age of 85 mothers with children aged under 5 referred to the NSPCC was

23 compared with the national average of 28. These studies, however, are all on a small scale. Some were carried out without control groups and different definitions of abuse were used. These factors make comparisons and generalizations very difficult. By contrast, Gil's (1970) sample of 1380 cases of reported abuse in the USA in the late 1960s led him to state that the age distribution of parents did 'not support the observation of many earlier studies of physically abused children and their families, according to which the parents tend to be extremely young' (Gil 1970: 110). Figures from the NSPCC suggested that such a view was still valid in the late 1980s (see Creighton and Noyes 1989: 16). The findings about age and physical abuse are not, therefore, consistent enough to provide clear connections and there is, as a result, need for care with their interpretation. It may be convenient to associate child abuse with young parenthood. However, the evidence is not nearly strong enough to have much predictive value, even in association with other factors considered indicative of risk.

Sexual abuse

There has been little emphasis placed on the age of adult sexual abuse perpetrators. By and large, fathers (and father substitutes) who sexually abuse children within the family are likely to be older than physically abusing parents because in most cases the age of the victim is higher (see pp. 124–5). However, the age of the abuser is not generally considered to be an important issue in sexual abuse, except where the perpetrator is a child or adolescent.

Abuse by adolescents and children

Abuse of younger children by adolescents has been the focus of much attention by researchers. Straus *et al.* (1980) estimated that over 19 million children a year (nearly one-third of the total child population of the USA) engaged in abusively violent acts against a sibling. They found that the violence was usually inflicted by older children on younger, that it decreased with age and, surprisingly, that aggression of this kind was only slightly more characteristic of boys (83 per cent) than girls (73 per cent).

Masson and Erooga (1999) estimate that between 25 and 33 per cent of all alleged sexual abuse involves young (mainly adolescent) perpetrators. Some studies (Abel *et al.* 1985) have found that as many as half of all convicted child sexual abusers started to commit sexual offences in adolescence or earlier.

Fehrenbach *et al.* (1986) estimated from a study of adolescent sex offenders that 95 per cent were male, that 19 per cent had been sexually abused themselves, that the bulk of their victims were known to them and that one-third were relatives. Burton *et al.* (1997) found that 79 per cent of a large sample of sexually aggressive children aged 12 and under were male. In this sample 72 per cent of the children had themselves already been sexually abused.

Johnson (1989) carried out a study of 13 female child perpetrators, aged between 4 and 12. Her main findings were, first, that these girls had all been severely sexually abused over long periods of time and, second, that most of their victims were members of their own families. Fehrenbach and Monastersky (1988) studied 28 female adolescents charged with rape or indecent liberties. They found that 20 of these had been either physically or sexually abused themselves and that most of the abuse they perpetrated took place when they were baby-sitting. While these two studies should remind us that girls sexually abuse children as well as boys, it should be noted that such abuse is primarily perpetrated by males.

Most of the above studies do not differentiate between intrafamilial and extrafamilial abuse. Adler and Schutz (1995) focused specifically on sibling incest, the dynamics and characteristics of which are in many ways more complex than in the case of extrafamilial abuse.

Poverty, race and child abuse

Physical abuse

Partly because of a traditional focus on individual and psychological factors in the understanding of child abuse, there has been less direct attention paid to the association between broader social factors, such as poverty and class, and child abuse. However, as we saw in Chapter 4, connections between social exclusion and child abuse are currently being explored more fully in Britain. That child protectionists have not paid more attention to the impact of social factors is strange because nearly all studies of official reports and most research surveys demonstrate a strong correlation between poverty and physical abuse and neglect. Gil (1970) found that between 80 and 90 per cent of parents of 1380 children who were officially reported to have been physically abused in the USA were in the lower social classes, with high dependency on public assistance benefits. Straus *et al.* (1980) found that blue-collar workers were more likely to punish physically and abuse their children. In Britain, Becker and Macpherson (1988) found that 90 per cent of referrals for child abuse in Strathclyde in the late 1980s involved children in families dependent on state benefits.

More recent research has shown that 95 per cent of children on child protection registers are from poor families (DoH 1995).

Nevertheless, it has been argued that child abuse is a cross-class phenomenon and that the high proportions of lower-class families being suspected of such abuse result from the fact that they are more open to state surveillance. This is because of their need for state resources, application for which is at the cost of reduced privacy and independence. From this point of view, the official figures merely demonstrate that the children of the poor who are being abused are more likely to be spotted than those in the higher social classes.

Children from non-white families are over-represented in official reports of child abuse in the USA. Gil (1970) found that one-third of all his sample cases were children from non-white families. At the time, such families constituted 15 per cent of the total population. Lauderdale *et al.* (1980) found that black families were also most likely to be reported for child abuse in the state of Texas. Incidence studies provide a mixed picture. Straus *et al.* (1980) found no difference between the rates of severe violence employed in black and white families in 1975. However, Hampton *et al.* (1989) found that such violence had increased in black families in the period between then and 1985, whereas for white families there had been a decline in its incidence. Burgdorff (1981) found that, compared with poor white families, poor black families were less abusive to their children.

Data regarding race and child protection have not yet been collected by government departments in Britain and very few studies check their samples for ethnicity. Hyman (1978) reported that 14 per cent of her sample of cases referred to the NSPCC had black fathers. Creighton and Noyes (1989), however, stressed that the overwhelming majority of the children registered by the NSPCC between 1983 and 1987 were from white European ethnic backgrounds. Generally the amount of hard information is meagre. One would expect black children to be over-represented in child abuse statistics, partly because their families are more open to surveillance as a result of figuring highly among indices of deprivation (Brown 1984) and partly because cultural misunderstanding and the operation of both institutional and direct racism may have increased the chances of suspicions of abuse in black families being confirmed.

Sexual abuse

Most incidence studies of child sexual abuse point to its existence among all strata of society. Finkelhor *et al.* (1986) argue that class, ethnic and regional factors do not seem to affect the incidence of sexual abuse of children in the USA. In a national survey held in 1985, the only exceptions to this were boys of English or Scandinavian

heritage, who were at higher risk than those from other ethnic groupings (Finkelhor *et al.* 1990). The MORI Poll survey in Britain found
that 'there are no significant differences between the abused, non-
abused and refused-to-answer groups with regard to social class and
area of residence' (Baker and Duncan 1985: 459).

However, most reported child sexual abuse is located disproportionately among poorer families. Ben-Tovim *et al.* (1988) kept rough figures
on families seen at Great Ormond Street Hospital between 1982 and
1986. Only 8 per cent of the fathers were employed in non-manual
occupations. The bulk of families coming to the notice of the NSPCC
as a result of child sexual abuse were from the poorer classes (Creighton
and Noyes 1989: 18–19). More recent studies (see DoH 1995) have
lent support to these findings, as has evidence from the USA (Finkelhor
1993). The arguments that apply to physical abuse and neglect regarding state surveillance of the poorer classes seem also to apply to
sexual abuse. Finkelhor was unequivocal about the implications of
the disparity of findings between research study and officially reported
statistics: 'professionals need to be cautioned against using incor-
rect, class-biased stereotypes, and that mechanisms for detecting, and
incentives for reporting cases from higher social classes need to be
strengthened' (Finkelhor 1993: 68).

There is little relevant information available on ethnicity and officially reported sexual abuse in Britain. It is unlikely that black families
will be over-represented in this category, because (as was stressed in
Chapter 4) there is a probability that cultural ignorance and stereotyp-
ing may lead to less intervention in this area rather than more (Stubbs
1989). In the USA black families are not over-represented in reports of
such abuse in comparison with the findings from epidemiological
studies (Finkelhor 1993).

Parents who have been abused themselves

The issue of the intergenerational transmission of abuse is a thorny
one indeed (see Kaufman and Zigler 1987, 1989). There are considerable
methodological problems in demonstrating linkages between behaviours over generations. At the level of common sense, the argument
that abused parents are more likely than non-abused parents to harm
their own children seems to have some credibility. However, it is
important to know whether this view is supported by empirical evidence and, if it is, then to what extent. Attention needs to be paid
to the discontinuities as well as the continuities. Knowledge of the
circumstances in which abused parents do not abuse their own children is of as much importance to child protection professionals as
that of the circumstances in which they do.

Physical abuse

Steele and Pollock (1974) interviewed 60 parents who had physically maltreated their children and found that they had all been abused themselves as children. Their definition of what constituted abuse for these parents was, however, very wide-ranging and included being subjected to 'intensive, pervasive and continual demands' from their own parents.

Oliver (1985), using official records, uncovered 147 families out of a population of 200,000 in north Wiltshire where abuse of children had happened in successive generations. However, the potential usefulness of this study is diminished by the fact that we are not told how many of the parents who were abused themselves in the first generation did not go on to abuse their own children.

Jayaratne (1977), using Gil's (1970) relatively low transmission rate findings (14 per cent in the case of mothers and 7 per cent in the case of fathers), argued against the intergenerational hypothesis. Cicchetti and Aber (1980) argued that the hypothesis has been overstated and that situational and interactional factors within the family are more telling indicators than the history of the parents.

Hunter and Kilstrom (1979) conducted an important study on this subject (particularly with respect to methodological issues). They interviewed 282 parents of new-born children admitted to a regional intensive care nursery for premature and ill infants. Of these parents, 49 (17 per cent) had themselves been abused. At follow-up a year later, nine of these had abused their children. Only one child from the rest of the sample had been abused. Thus the intergenerational rate in this prospective study was 18 per cent. However, if the ten children who were abused had become the subject of a retrospective study, it would have been found that 90 per cent of their parents had been abused and this could give an exaggerated impression of the extent of intergenerational abuse.

Egeland (1988) followed up over a period of 12 years 267 women considered before the birth of their first child to be at some risk of abuse, and found that there was an intergenerational transmission rate of abuse of about one-third. Perhaps more importantly, he also looked for factors that improved parents' chances of avoiding repetition of the abuse that they had experienced, and identified two: the development of satisfying personal relationships and social networks; and an ability to verbalize and be open about their own experiences.

The findings of this study are supported by those of an earlier study by Straus (1979). Making an estimate from the 1975 intrafamilial violence incidence study, carried out by him and his colleagues, he concluded that the rate of all types of intergenerational abuse varied between 25 and 35 per cent. He found that there was more risk for the child if the parents had been ill-treated, but that the majority of ill-treated children do not become abusive parents.

It is worth noting an issue raised earlier: that all these studies focus almost entirely on transmission of violence and abuse through mothers whereas, to the best of our knowledge, men are responsible for at least half of all physical abuse. There is very little research into the antecedents of male adults who physically abuse.

Sexual abuse

The picture is only slightly better in this respect with regard to sexual abuse. Despite the fact that males are responsible for nearly all such abuse, there is still considerable focus on women as the key link between sexual abuse over two generations. Goodwin *et al.* (1981) found that 24 per cent of mothers of abused children had had prior incest experiences compared with 3 per cent of a control group. Faller (1989) found that nearly half the mothers of a sample of 154 sexually abused children either had experienced or knew of sexual abuse in their own families of origin. This study is particularly useful in that it also checked the experiences of the male offenders in these cases; nearly 40 per cent of them had also experienced or knew of sexual abuse in their families as children.

Studies of male perpetrators of sexual abuse who have been imprisoned show relatively high proportions of these men having been sexually abused themselves as children. Groth and Burgess (1979) found that 32 per cent of a group of 106 child molesters reported some form of sexual trauma in childhood. Yet of the 274 cases seen by Ben-Tovim *et al.* (1988), only five of the perpetrators had been abused themselves. The differences may be explained by the fact that these studies were looking at two different types of sexual abuser: persistent offenders who are a danger to many children outside their families and those who have focused their attentions on the children immediately available to them within the family.[4] As we saw earlier, high proportions of young sexual abusers have been sexually abused; Johnson (1988) found that 49 per cent of child perpetrators of sexual abuse had themselves been abused and (as has been already stated) young female sexual offenders also studied by her were all found to have been sexually abused.

There is clearly some intergenerational linking between sexual abuse. It seems to be roughly in the same proportions as for physical abuse and neglect. However, the form of transmission is complex. This is partly due to the focus of the research studies. There is little attention paid to intrafamilial male adult abusers and, therefore, little information about them. Faller's (1989) study is an exception to this. There is more information about persistent child abusers and about the abuse experienced by mothers of children who are sexually abused. The focus on the latter seems to implicate such women in the abuse of their children. It is interesting to note the rarity of sexual abuse by women given the extent of abuse they experience, whereas the opposite seems to be true of men.

It is worth noting that although sexual and physical abuse have been considered separately, several of the studies point to sexual abusers having themselves experienced both forms of abuse in childhood. Studies of families where organized abuse has been found, point, in the worst cases, to multiple types of abuse over two and more generations (see Bibby 1996).

The topic of intergenerational transmission of abuse is clearly a problematic one. It has been argued that focus on this issue is pessimistic as far as those who have been abused are concerned. It can also, from another point of view, be seen to be over-deterministic, taking away individuals' responsibilities for their own actions. That continuities exist is not in dispute but, as Straus pointed out in the late 1970s, there are more pertinent questions to be asked:

> The time has come for the intergenerational myth to be put aside and for researchers to cease arguing 'Do abused children become abusive parents?' and ask, instead, 'Under what conditions is the transmission of abuse likely to occur?'
>
> (Straus 1979: 191)

Family structure and child abuse

There is considerable current concern about the changing shape of the family and the effect that it may be having on child care practices and children's behaviour (see Fox-Harding 1996). Official statistics show that lone parenthood has increased dramatically since the 1960s as has divorce – one-third of all marriages now end in divorce and large numbers of children live in reconstituted families.[5] Two facets of family structure have been particularly considered by child abuse researchers: lone parenthood and step-parenting (particularly with regard to sexual abuse).

Lone-parent families

In the USA official figures in 1981 showed that 43 per cent of children reported for all kinds of abuse came from single-female household heads and 5 per cent from single-male household heads, the national percentage for all such households being 17 (National Center on Child Abuse and Neglect 1981). Creighton and Noyes (1989) found that one-quarter of all children registered for physical abuse by the NSPCC in England and Wales between 1983 and 1987 lived in lone-parent families. Nearly half of those registered for neglect, over half of those registered for failure to thrive and one-third of those registered for emotional abuse also lived in lone-parent households.

With regard to physical abuse and neglect, Sack *et al.* (1985) carried out a study of 802 adults in Oregon and found the prevalence of abuse to be twice as high in single-parent households as in those with two parents. Gelles (1989), using data from two national incidence studies of violence in the family, came to the conclusion that lone-parent families were no more likely than two-parent families to use violence overall, but that they were more likely to use severe and very severe violence, particularly in the case of the single male parent. Creighton and Noyes (1989) found somewhat surprisingly that one-fifth of children registered for sexual abuse came from lone-female headed homes. On the face of it, one would expect such children to be safer from abuse by males.

Overall both official reports and survey findings concur: children in lone-parent families are more at risk of all forms of abuse and neglect than their counterparts in two-parent families. To what extent this is the case is not clear; Gelles's (1989) estimate is much lower than that of Sack *et al.* (1985). In addition, these rather bald statistics do not tell us anything about the dynamics or processes that might help to account for this variation in abuse rates between these two family types. Clearly economic stress is likely to be an important factor. The high percentage of neglect cases among lone-parent families shown up in the NSPCC figures could also point to this. Issues surrounding the control of children and social isolation could also play a part. With regard to sexual abuse, Finkelhor *et al.* (1986) argue that children in lone-female headed households could be exposed to a greater number of male adult figures than those in two-parent households and that this could place them at statistically greater risk of being sexually abused.

All this paints a rather negative picture of lone-parenting. The advantages of such families should also be taken into account, such as the potential for less interpersonal conflict between parents, a factor which has been associated with emotional abuse. There is need for much more research into the impact of lone-parenting (benefits and costs) on child-rearing in general.

Step-parents

There is not a great deal of available information on the impact of step-parenting on physical abuse and neglect. Creighton and Noyes (1989) found that 32 per cent of physically abused children lived with one natural parent (mainly female) and one substitute parent (mainly male). The percentages for other forms of abuse were as follows: neglect 15 per cent, failure to thrive 11 per cent and emotional abuse 36 per cent. Reconstituted families are thus well over-represented in these abuse statistics, but there has been little follow-up research as to why this is the case or into the process of abuse in such families.

However, there seems to be much fascination with the issue of whether blood-tie parents are more likely to abuse their children sexually than non-blood-tie relatives and more research into this topic as a result. Of the cases seen by Ben-Tovim *et al.* (1988) between 1982 and 1986, 46 per cent of the perpetrators were natural parents and 27 per cent step-parents (nearly all male). Of 198 paternal offenders studied by Gordon and Creighton (1988), 46 per cent were non-natal fathers and 54 per cent were birth fathers. Russell (1984) found from her sample of 930 women that 17 per cent (one in six) of those who had had a stepfather as a principal figure during their childhood had been sexually abused by him and that the comparable figures for biological fathers was 2 per cent (one in forty). In addition she found that stepfathers were more likely to commit seriously abusive acts. It seems to be the case, therefore, that children are more at risk of being sexually abused by a step-parent or parent-substitute than by their natural parents.

Two caveats need to be borne in mind. First, there is a danger of assuming that all step-parents present a risk to children. This is clearly not true. Even using Russell's (1984) high figures of stepfather abuse, five out of six step-fathers do not sexually abuse their step-children. Second, as Russell herself commented, there are 'no grounds whatsoever for considering sexual abuse by step-fathers as less serious than sexual abuse by biological fathers' (Russell 1986: 16). There is clearly a need for more broad-based research into the impact of family structure on children in reconstituted families and, as with lone-parent families, there is need for attention to be paid to positive features and adaptations as well as to negative consequences.

The psychological capacities of those who abuse

This section looks, first, at whether mental illness plays a part in the causation of physical child abuse and, second, at the association between such abuse and the intellectual capacities of parents. Research into the psychological make-up of child sexual abusers will then be considered.

Physical abuse and mental illness

Mainstream thinking about linkages between physical child abuse and neglect and mental health issues has been fairly limited. The view held by early child abuse pioneers such as Steele and Pollock (1974) was that, in the main, women (there is very little reference to men) who abused their children were not mentally ill. They were considered to have problems with parenting linked to psychological incapacities to nurture and care for their babies and children. Only a small number of parents were thought to be experiencing mental illness (see Kempe and Kempe 1978) and in these cases it was considered unsafe to consider rehabilitation; it is notable that the term 'psychotic' is used to describe these cases. Greenland (1987) found that less than nine parents in the 100 cases where child deaths had occurred in Ontario were suffering from mental illnesses, but they were all of a severe psychotic nature. Straus *et al.* (1980) attributed less than 10 per cent of all types of family violence to mental illness.

There are some studies that have taken a broader definition of mental illness and, as a result, have demonstrated a closer association between such illness and physical child abuse. Hyman (1978) found that, in 21 out of the 85 cases (25 per cent) she studied, psychiatric illness had been diagnosed in the mothers. Oliver (1985) found that 50 out of 147 mothers (34 per cent) had been treated psychiatrically for depression, as had seven of the fathers (5 per cent). Smith (1975) found that three-quarters of the mothers and two-thirds of the fathers in his study of 214 parents had 'abnormal personalities', but only a very few had been formally diagnosed as mentally ill. Research carried out by Falkov (1996) into Part 8 Reviews of child deaths and serious abuse found that mental illness (maternal and paternal) was evident in 32 of the 100 cases.

It may be the case that there are some forms of psychological state, such as depression, whose effects and influence are underestimated as contributory factors to the physical abuse and neglect of children. Brown and Harris (1978) associated depression in working-class women with a variety of poor environmental factors. There are also links between men's violence to women and depression (see Kelly 1988). The role of depression seems to have been underplayed in thought about and research into child abuse. The female carers of several children who have been the subject of public inquiries, such as Christine Mason (Lambeth, Lewisham and Southwark 1989), Beatrice Henry (Lambeth 1987) and Rosemary Koseda (Hillingdon 1986), have all been described as showing symptoms of depression.[6] It should also be noted that research in Britain (Farmer and Owen 1995; Thoburn *et al.* 1995) found relatively high rates of depression (and of physical illnesses) among families undergoing child protection investigations.

Some family violence researchers are very keen to dissociate forms of abuse from mental illness on the grounds that such violence should not be seen to be the product of abnormal behavioural states, but rather the acts of sane people (Gelles and Cornell 1985). Roberts (1988: 46) epitomizes this view: 'psychiatric labels seem unjustified when so many practitioners are convinced that the potential for child abuse is within us all, given a sufficient number of stressful circumstances'. There is also a danger that focusing on the role of depression in child abuse could serve to place even more emphasis on women. Nevertheless, this seems to be an area of concern that merits further consideration.

Physical abuse and parents with learning difficulties

There has been only a small amount of research into parents with learning difficulties who abuse their children. Some early studies pointed to a very strong connection between low intelligence and child abuse. Rates drawn from samples by Young (1964) and Smith (1975) were as high as 50 per cent. Such findings have not, however, been replicated in more recent studies. Creighton and Noyes (1989) found that 10 per cent of mothers and 5 per cent of fathers of children on registers had attended special schools. While this is a much lower rate than those suggested by the earlier studies, it is still well above the national level. Thus there is evidence of a significant correlation between learning disability and officially reported child abuse.

There are, however, several factors that could account for this association, the most obvious being that the heightened concern that exists with regard to people with learning difficulties bringing up their own children results in their child care practices being exposed to greater scrutiny than those of parents of normal intelligence. Care should be taken not to see all people with learning difficulties as a homogeneous group with similar characteristics. They do share some common problems, but these stem mainly from their potential for being undervalued and exploited by others.

Research that demonstrates the circumstances in which parents with learning difficulties abuse their children is more useful than research that simply demonstrates correlation rates between low intelligence and child abuse. The study by Tymchuk and Andron (1990) is a good example of this. They compared two small groups of low IQ mothers, half of whom had a history of abuse or neglect of their own children and half who had not. The former in fact had higher IQs than the latter. The important difference seemed to be the degree of support they had received as pregnant women and parents. The women who had neglected their children had received far less support than the non-neglecters.

Sexual abuse

There has been little linkage between particular psychological characteristics and child sexual abuse. There has been much more emphasis on interactive rather than individualistic factors than in the case of physical abuse and neglect. There has been no research linking mental illness with sexual abuse. Traditionally, incest has been linked to families of low intelligence, but there is little research evidence to show this to be the case.

Finkelhor *et al.* (1986), however, raised several important questions about the personality characteristics of those who sexually abuse children, such as why a person would find relating to a child sexually gratifying and congruent; why a person would be sexually aroused by a child; why a person would be blocked in efforts to obtain sexual and emotional gratification from more normally approved sources; and, finally, why a person would not be affected by societal taboos. Research into these questions and others relating to the psychological make-up of those who sexually abuse children is urgently needed. To some extent, these issues are being taken up by those involved in sex offender treatment programmes (see Morrison *et al.* 1994). Considerable understanding has been gained of the psychological processes involved in targeting, grooming and abusing children. The focus of these programmes is largely on cognitive processes and getting offenders to acknowledge and take responsibility for their actions. There is little evidence of psychiatric illness being a factor in material emanating from these programmes.

Other factors associated with those who abuse children

There are many other factors associated with those who abuse children. In this section, five other areas will be briefly addressed: alcohol and drugs; social isolation; partner problems and wife abuse; criminality; and pregnancy, prematurity, bonding and other neonatal problems.

Alcohol and drugs

Alcohol has been closely linked with child abuse from the early days of the NSPCC at the time when the Temperance movement had a high profile. It is still cited as a contributory factor to physical child abuse (Browne and Saqi 1988). However, Orme and Rimmer (1981) in their review of research into the connection between alcoholism and physical child abuse up to that date pointed out that assessing the value of the different studies was difficult because of the problems of achieving common definitions of the two phenomena. They came to this conclusion: 'The most striking finding that emerged from our study was that there was not adequate empirical evidence to support an association between alcoholism and child abuse' (Orme and Rimmer 1981: 285).

Alcohol misuse has a higher association with child neglect. Studies in the USA point to as many as half of all families known to the public welfare system being affected by alcohol or drug misuse (see Curtis and McCullogh 1993). Alcohol misuse clearly heightens concerns among professionals about the ability of parents to care properly for their children, even if a direct linkage with physical abuse remains unproved.

Another related concern has been that of the impact of excessive alcohol misuse on the unborn baby (foetal alcohol syndrome) which can include severe mental retardation and still births (see Collins 1990).

There has been little empirical research into the connection between sexual abuse and alcoholism. La Fontaine (1990: 100) quotes Maisch (1973): 'It would be a mistake to deduce from suitable cases a direct, specific causal connection between alcohol and incest.'

There is growing concern about the connection between drug misuse and child ill-treatment. There are few hard data available in Britain. Dore *et al.* (1995) pointed to very high rates of drug misuse among substantiated child mistreatment cases in the USA. As with alcohol, it is not clear from these figures whether drug misuse is associated more with physical abuse or neglect. It is probably the latter. In other words, there is an increasing likelihood that parental drug misuse will be seen as a major risk factor in terms of the care of children (see Murphy *et al.* 1991). Drug misuse is also a concern in regard to foetal abuse (see Parker *et al.* 1988).

More detailed information on this subject is clearly needed with much greater attention being placed on how and in what circumstances children are placed at risk by parental misuse of drugs and alcohol, in order to avoid assuming an automatic linkage between substance misuse and abuse of children.

Social isolation

The connection between social isolation and child abuse has been persuasively argued by Garbarino (1982) and Polansky *et al.* (1979), among others. This topic will be discussed as a causal explanation of child abuse in more detail in Chapter 8. Smith (1975) found that 49 per cent of his sample of abusing parents had no opportunities for having a break from the child, as opposed to 26 per cent in his control group. They had no contact with parents, relatives, neighbours or friends. Several other studies of physical abuse and neglect report similar findings (Skinner and Castle 1969; Giovannoni and Billingsley 1970). However, the value of these studies is limited. First, they do not employ common definitions of social isolation. Second, they do not measure the quality of contacts. An individual may have many familial and social contacts, but these may not be supportive or alleviate the stresses of child care. Third, they do not help us understand the impact of social isolation on abuse, whether it causes it or is an effect of it. There is an assumption that social isolation is a causal factor, but families may isolate themselves to prevent the discovery of abuse (see Reder *et al.* 1993), or become isolated because they are neglecting their children. Therefore, although there is a rough association between certain forms of abuse and social isolation, there is a need for more detailed research into the way in which these variables interact.

More recent studies (Seagull 1987; Coohey 1996) have paid more attention to defining social isolation. Coohey (1996) lists three important variables that should be measured in assessing the impact of isolation: the number of network contacts, the amount of received support and the parents' perception of that support. It is notable that both she and Seagull (1987) found a higher correlation between social isolation and neglect than for any other form of abuse.

Partner problems and wife abuse

Lukianowicz (1971), in an early study, pointed to an association between physically abusive parents and poor marital relationships. Ben-Tovim *et al.* (1988) found that half the perpetrators of child sexual abuse and two-thirds of their partners considered that they had relationship problems. Creighton and Noyes (1989) found that the stress factor that was ranked as most severe for all registered children was the 'marital problems' of their parents. However, the usefulness of this aspect of knowledge is open to question. First, there are problems involved in assessing the quality of relationships. Second, there are many adults with children who have relationship problems and do not abuse their children. Third, abuse of children may take place with no apparent conflict between its adult carers.[7] Fourth, the term 'marital or partner problems' could include a whole host of behaviours that may not be equally important. For instance, it could include constant verbal rows and violent physical assaults. Certainly, as a predictive tool, this aspect of knowledge is fairly useless.

A more fruitful area of study in relation to the quality of parental relationships and the connection with child abuse is that which deals with domestic violence. Brekke (1987) has pointed to a connection between wife abuse and child physical abuse, and Truesdell *et al.* (1986) has pointed to a similar linkage in relation to sexual abuse. More recent research (Farmer and Owen 1995) has reaffirmed the connection between physical abuse of children and wife abuse, and the growing concerns about the impact of wife abuse on a child's emotional development has already been referred to (see Mullender and Morley 1994). Mayhew *et al.* (1993) found that there were 530,000 assaults on women by men each year in Britain and that in 90 per cent of these cases children were in either the same or an adjacent room at the time of the assault. Studies such as these are important in raising public awareness and developing greater determination to tackle wife abuse at a broader societal level, which in turn should have an impact on the protection of children in families where male violence to women partners exists.

However, as with much of the other research referred to in this chapter, there is a pressing need for studies which go beyond correlations and explore in greater depth the dynamics of the family processes where child abuse and wife abuse coexist, so that child protection intervention in these circumstances can be better informed (see Coohey and Braun 1997).

Criminality

Previous history of child ill-treatment on the part of an adult is considered to be an important indicator of risk with regard to children living with them. Creighton and Noyes (1989) demonstrated that there was an increase in the numbers of parents with records for offences against children figuring in child protection registrations between 1983 and 1987. In many of the cases that were the subject of public inquiries, parents, particularly fathers, had been previously convicted of offences against children. However, there has been little systematic research into recidivism rates with regard to physical abuse of children.

Somewhat more attention has been paid to recidivism rates among child sexual abusers. Furby et al. (1989) in a review of studies found the rate to be as high as 56 per cent in some and that this was regardless of whether offenders receive specific treatment or not. Abel et al. (1987) and Elliott et al. (1995) show that the worst extrafamilial offenders may have hundreds of victims. Care has to be taken not to extrapolate findings such as these to all those who have sexually abused children, in that the studies reviewed focus largely on the extreme end of the spectrum. It would be useful to know, if there are sexual offenders who do not reoffend, what their characteristics are and the circumstances of their offending.

As we saw in Chapter 4, there was an escalation of concerns about child sexual abusers in Britain in the 1990s, particularly as a result of the discovery of large numbers of cases of institutional abuse. This led to the tightening of measures in the selection of residential staff (see Warner 1992) and to new legislation, the 1997 Sex Offenders Act, empowering the police to monitor and track sex offenders released from prison and to pass on information about them to those deemed to need to know.

Some studies have pointed to correlations between general criminality and child abuse. Oliver (1985), in his study of 147 families who had abused children over two generations, found a considerable degree of general criminality among his sample, but only a small amount of such criminality was associated with child abuse. Correlations of this kind tell us little other than about the type of family whose children come under closest scrutiny from the state. There seems to be no logical reason why general criminality should have any particular connection with child abuse.

There is a need for a good deal of caution in using previous history of child abuse on the part of adults as an indicator of their children being at risk. Our current state of knowledge is very limited. At present it suggests, first, that there is a need to investigate such circumstances, and second, that care should be taken not to assume that 'once an offender, always an offender'. In relation to sexual abuse, particularly extrafamilial abuse, our knowledge of offending behaviour points in the opposite direction. As we have already seen, there are high levels of recidivism.

Pregnancy, prematurity, bonding and other neonatal problems

Greenland (1987) points out that several studies in the 1960s and 1970s found a correlation between child abuse and pregnancy. Elmer (1977) found that nine of her sample of 20 abusive mothers were pregnant at the time the abuse was referred. It should not be construed from this that all pregnant women are a threat to their other children. This is clearly not the case. The message of findings such as these is that pregnancy can create extra stress on parents, knowledge of which may be crucial to ongoing work with families where children are already considered to be at risk.

Peri-natal and neonatal difficulties have received arguably more attention than any other potential causal factor in the study of child abuse. The general view adopted by researchers in this field is that where there are problems at birth, such as prematurity, which result in early separation of mother and child, there is a potential for poor mother–child relationships, rejection and abuse. Lynch and Roberts (1977) reported that use of a checklist, including significant separation from the child after birth and concerns reported by midwives about mothers' early responses to their babies, was an effective predictor of future care and potential abuse. Murphy *et al.* (1981) retrospectively studied 80 cases of children abused in the Cardiff area and found that, compared with controls, more had been born pre-term and were of lower birth weight. In the USA, Benedict and White (1985) studied over 500 cases in a similar way and also associated prematurity, low birth weights and longer stays in hospital around birth with children who were later abused. On the other hand, Leventhal *et al.* (1984) found no relationship between prematurity, low birth weight and abuse in a study of 117 abused children (with controls). There was a much closer correlation with young maternal age than with any other factor.

Most of the evidence, despite Leventhal *et al.*'s (1984) findings, points to a correlation between birth problems and later abuse and neglect. This does not mean, of course, that wherever these types of birth difficulties occur abuse will result. It means that the chances are higher. The research findings demonstrate the connections, but do not necessarily explain why they exist or the process whereby abuse results. Bonding difficulties have been most often cited as potential causal factors, that is mothers and children miss out on a crucial time for attachment to each other, which can set in train a set of events such as uncertain handling, problems in feeding and lack of mutual pleasure, leading ultimately to abuse. However, doubts have been raised about the crucial importance attached to immediate post-birth bonding (see Sluckin *et al.* 1983). Other factors could account for the correlation between neonatal difficulties and child abuse. First, looking after prematurely born and/or low birth weight children who generally require more attention and care is likely to put carers under extreme stress. Second, it is probable that the majority of the mothers in these studies who were experiencing peri-natal difficulties were from poor backgrounds (see Dingwall 1989). Inadequate material resources for looking after young babies are probably an additional major factor in the quality of care that is provided.[8] Much medical-based research tends to underplay such social concerns.

As with most of the other research in this chapter, the focus of studies of neonatal bonding problems is on the mother. This is a major weakness. There needs to be more attention paid to the involvement (or lack of involvement) of fathers in early child care. Some studies have suggested that the lack of early bonding between fathers and children could be a contributory factor in the causation of child sexual abuse (see Parker and Parker 1986).

Who is abused

All children are potentially vulnerable to abuse by those adults who look after them through childhood because they are dependent on them for all aspects of physical and emotional protection and care. Most children are not mistreated by their parents because protective behaviour is considered natural and instinctive (Bowlby 1971). However, a great deal of effort has been expended on trying to predict where breakdowns in this normal protective behaviour are likely to occur, by focusing on the characteristics and circumstances of children who are abused as well as on those of their parents. Clearly there are factors common to both, and in the section on who abuses (pp. 103–23), those associated with parents, such as their own experiences of abuse, their psychological state and the quality of their marital or partner relationships, have been considered and do not need to be reviewed again here. Finkelhor and Korbin (1988), writing from an international perspective, but with an eye to poorer countries in the southern hemisphere, point out that the following children are most vulnerable to abuse and neglect:

- children with inferior health status
- children who are deformed or handicapped (though in a few societies they are protected by a special status)
- female children
- children born in unusual, stigmatized or difficult conditions
- excess or unwanted children
- children with disvalued traits and behaviours
- illegitimate children
- children born in situations of rapid economic change.

While such children are less obviously at risk in northern industrialized societies, they are still more vulnerable to abuse within these societies than those who do not share these characteristics. Many of the factors listed above have been considered in the first section of this chapter. The factors that remain to be discussed are age; gender; parent–child relationship problems; physical and mental disabilities; family size.

Age

Using Department of Health statistics for 1999, the age breakdown of children on child protection registers is set out in Table 7.1. The unborn category of children includes those about to be born to parents who have already seriously abused siblings and increasingly those due to be born to parents involved in substance misuse. Concerns about under 1-year-olds are largely in relation to physical abuse and neglect. Children in this age group are more likely to be registered for these reasons than those in older age groups, reflecting the concerns created by their particular vulnerability.

The pattern is reversed for sexual abuse, the age group most likely to be registered under this category being those aged 10–15. Using figures from prevalence studies, Finkelhor (1993) found that in the USA there was a dramatic increase in risk for sexual abuse at age 10, preceded by some rise in vulnerability about ages 6–7. One must be

Table 7.1 The age of children placed on child protection registers during the year ending 31 March 1999

Unborn	300
Under 1	3,000
1–4	9,700
5–9	9,700
10–15	8,600
16+	600
Total	31,900

Table 7.2 Child protection registrations during the year ending 31 March 1999 by gender

Boys	14,700
Girls	14,600
Unborn	800
Total	30,100

careful in using these figures not to assume that certain forms of abuse are confined to certain age ranges. Finkelhor (1993) also notes that children under 6 constitute at least 10 per cent of child sexual abuse victims in the USA (see also Hobbs and Wynne 1986; Macfarlane and Waterman 1986). The case of Stephen Menhenniot (DHSS 1978) provides a salutary reminder that physical abuse of young people can persist almost to adulthood.[9]

Gender

In the year ending 31 March 1999, there were 30,100 children placed on child protection registers; the gender breakdown is set out in Table 7.2. As can be seen, girls and boys are equally likely to be registered for child abuse. Boys are more exposed to physical abuse, neglect and emotional abuse than girls, as far as official intervention is concerned. Creighton and Noyes (1989) reported similar findings from the NSPCC register returns between 1983 and 1987. There seem to be no obvious reasons why this is the case. It could be speculated that, in the case of physical abuse, physical punishment of boys is more generally sanctioned as a means of control in our society than of girls and that this cultural norm leads to more excessive violence in their case. Girls are considerably more likely to be represented in official child sexual abuse registrations than boys. Finkelhor (1993) noted from the US scene that from prevalence studies boys constitute 29 per cent of sexual abuse victims whereas in official statistics they account for only 20 per cent.

Finkelhor and Korbin (1988) argued that in many societies throughout the world (India, for example) girls are more subjected to abuse because they are less valued for their economic utility. In western society, these economic factors do not apply.

Parent–child relationship problems

There has been a good deal written about the contribution of the child to his or her own abuse. This seems a strange and, on the face of it, somewhat offensive concept. However, there is some evidence to suggest that particular children are singled out for abuse. Family therapists, in particular, and behaviourists are interested in the dynamics of child abuse and why particular children are 'selected' for such abuse and not others. Children who are not wanted or who are considered to be the wrong sex by their parents are seen to be at greater risk (see Roberts *et al.* 1980). Friedrich and Boriskin (1976) listed a variety of factors associated with the child that may contribute to abuse taking place. These include prematurity and genetic differences, which make some children cuddlers and some not. The latter are seen to be more at risk because they do not 'reward' their parents.

> It would be fanciful to conclude that the special child is the sole contributor to abuse. But the opposite extreme, the all too prevalent notion that abuse is exclusively a function of a parental defect, seems equally specious.
>
> (Friedrich and Boriskin 1976: 288)

Once again, the dynamics of the situation need to be stressed. Much depends on the parent–child mix. As Belsky and Vondra (1989) so clearly put it:

> The undermining effect of a difficult child on parental functioning will be lessened when the parent has an abundance of personal psychological resources. Conversely, an easy-to-rear child can compensate for limited personal resources on the part of the parent in maintaining parental effectiveness.
>
> (Belsky and Vondra 1989: 188)

Turning to extrafamilial sexual abuse, including that which takes place in institutions, the following comments from Finkelhor seem pertinent here:

> First, a child is more vulnerable to abuse if the child's activities and contacts are inadequately supervised and monitored. Secondly, a child who is emotionally neglected or physically or psychologically abused, is also more vulnerable to the ploys of child molesters

who offer attention and affection, or even intimidation, to involve children in sexual contacts.

(Finkelhor 1993: 69)

Physical and mental disabilities

There is no doubt that children with physical and mental disabilities place additional child-rearing strains on families. It might be expected, therefore, that such children are more likely to be exposed to abuse and neglect. A review of US studies (White *et al.* 1987) came to the conclusion that there were linkages between children with physical disabilities and child abuse, but that the nature of the linkages was not clear (see also Westcott 1993).

Jaudes and Diamond (1985), using data from a study of 37 children with cerebral palsy, argued that it is necessary to disentangle abuse that causes disability from that inflicted on already disabled children. They concluded that as many as one-tenth of mental disabilities may be caused by abuse and that abuse of disabled children is relatively higher than abuse of the non-disabled population. Ammerman *et al.*'s (1989) study supported this view. Theringer *et al.* (1990) pointed out that children with mental handicaps are particularly vulnerable to sexual abuse and exploitation because of their relatively powerless position.

Benedict *et al.* (1990) provided a dissenting voice. However, the weight of the evidence is that disabled children are more vulnerable to abuse than their non-disabled counterparts. This view is further strengthened by the work of Marchant and Page (1992) which showed how communication problems are a major but not insurmountable barrier to enabling children with disabilities to disclose abuse.

We need to find out more about which disabled children in which situations are most at risk. Friedrich (1979), in a general study of parents with children with disabilities, found that marital satisfaction was the best overall predictor of coping. Such a finding obviously does not take into account the situation of lone parents. Nevertheless, the gist of the message is clear, namely that close support and help are important ingredients in bringing up all children and particularly those with disabilities.

Family size

Creighton (1984) and Creighton and Noyes (1989) found that families with four or more children figured disproportionately in cases registered by the NSPCC between 1977 and 1987. Just over 25 per cent of all registrations involved such families, yet at the time they constituted only 10 per cent of families with children in social classes IV and V.

Creighton and Noyes (1989) broke down the registrations by category of type of abuse for the years 1983 to 1987 and found that families with four or more children constituted just over one-third of all sexual abuse registrations and just under one-third of all neglect registrations. A related issue is that of the age gap between children. Some studies have found that there is a correlation between abuse and families with several children close in age (see Browne and Saqi 1988: 59–60). It must be concluded, therefore, that children in larger families with siblings close in age are statistically more at risk of abuse.

Concluding comments

The research studies considered in this chapter have all sought to answer the two questions of who abuses and who is abused, with the aim of pinpointing targets of prevention and intervention. As we have seen, there are weaknesses and biases in most of the research studies that to a large degree reduce their usefulness for practice. The main weaknesses of these studies have been repeatedly stressed.

They are, first, that they have focused too much on general correlations and not enough on particular details, so that we know, for example, that children living in reconstituted families are overall more at risk than those living with both natural parents. Yet we know little about the degree of risk, what factors exacerbate the risk or in what conditions reconstituted families do a good job of rearing children. These sorts of criticism apply to almost all of the factors that have been associated in the research studies with child abuse. The reason for this weakness lies in the mislaid emphasis on predicting and targeting the problem. There is a need to consider the hows and whys of child abuse as well. Second, many of the studies demonstrate gender-blindness and slip into the easy assumption that the mother is the key figure in the child abuse process. Again such a view does not do justice to the hows and whys of child abuse.

This does not completely invalidate the work that has been done, but stresses that it needs to be used in a careful and critical manner. Such research can, if used carefully, sensitize professionals to risk potential, but so far it provides a basic starting-point only.

Recommended reading

Ben-Tovim, A., Elton, A., Hildebrand, J., Tranter, M. and Vizard, E. (eds) (1988) *Child Sexual Abuse within the Family: Assessment and Treatment: The Work of the Great Ormond Street Team.* London: Wright.

Creighton, S. and Noyes, P. (1989) *Child Abuse Trends in England and Wales 1983–1987*. London: NSPCC.

Finkelhor, D. (1993) Epidemiological factors in the clinical identification of child sexual abuse, *Child Abuse and Neglect*, 17: 67–70.

Morrison, T., Erooga, M. and Beckett, R. (1994) *Sexual Offending Against Children: Assessment and Treatment of Male Abusers*. London: Routledge.

Reder, P., Duncan, S. and Gray, M. (1993) *Beyond Blame: Child Abuse Tragedies Revisited*. London: Routledge.

chapter **eight**

THE CAUSATION OF
CHILD ABUSE

Social workers and other professionals involved in the field of child abuse have generally been less concerned about why such abuse happens than they have about the type of person who abuses and the type of child who is most vulnerable to abuse. This is probably because the latter two questions seem to have a more direct impact on prediction and prevention (if we can identify those most likely to be at risk, then we can do something about it). The question of why child abuse happens is not considered so directly significant to the day-to-day practicalities of child protection work. Such an inquiry has traditionally been seen to be more the province of theorists than of practitioners. This state of affairs is understandable, given the increased volume of child protection work and the pressures on front-line workers not to make mistakes. However, endeavouring to understand why abuse of children takes place serves three main functions. It gives a greater sense of control to the worker over events that may otherwise seem inexplicable, it gives a sense of direction for ongoing work or treatment (whichever term is preferred) and it informs those responsible for policy-making in this field. For these reasons, understanding why abuse has happened has a very important contribution to make to child protection work.

A broad range of theoretical perspectives has been brought to bear on the aetiology of child abuse. They derive from diverse sources, survey the problem at different levels and, as a consequence, do not necessarily complement each other. Indeed there is a good deal of conflict and disagreement between adherents of different approaches, creating problems that until recently have not been constructively addressed. There is evidence of a move towards a resolution of these issues with the development of integrative approaches, which go some way towards combining the various perspectives to provide more comprehensive but also, inevitably, more complex explanatory accounts (see Garbarino 1977; Belsky 1980).

Overviews of causation theories tend to categorize them in different ways (see Sweet and Resick 1979; Ostbloom and Crase 1980). However, there seem to be three main groups of perspective:

- *psychological theories:* those that focus on the instinctive and psychological qualities of individuals who abuse
- *social psychological theories:* those that focus on the dynamics of the interaction between abuser, child and immediate environment
- *sociological perspectives:* those that emphasize social and political conditions as the most important reason for the existence of child abuse.

This categorization will be used as the structure for this chapter. In addition, consideration will be given to attempts to combine these perspectives to provide a more holistic picture.

Psychological theories

In this section consideration will be given to the contributions of the discipline of biology, attachment theory, psychodynamic theory, learning theory and cognitive approaches.

Biology and child abuse

There has been little direct application of principles drawn from the biological sciences to the understanding of child abuse among humans. Nevertheless, biological theory does underlie some approaches, particularly those of attachment theory and the psychodynamic perspective; it is has been argued, notably by sociobiologists, that Darwinian theories, such as natural selection and the survival of the fittest, have something to offer our understanding of child abuse.[1] Reite (1987) put forward the view that there are many factors common to human child care and neglect and that of animals:

> Human and non-human primates share a substantial common evolutionary history, and many of the behavioral systems we are talking about, including perhaps much of that underlying social attachment are likely biologically determined to a significant degree.
> (Reite 1987: 354)

He points out that animals abuse their young in circumstances where there are aberrations or disturbances in early mother–infant attachment, and where environmental stresses such as overcrowding or lack of social support prevail. In a similar vein, other writers have drawn some comparisons between certain types of child abuse and what is termed 'the culling process' among animals, whereby the weakest in the litter are neglected in times of food shortage (Barash 1981).

Sociobiologists have in a very general way applied these principles to the issue of step-parenting and substitute-parenting and child abuse. Some non-genetic parents in the animal world have been noted to be very cruel to infants. Hrdy (1977) found that in one species of monkey, males seeking to mate with females already with litters, but with no male protector, killed the young. The explanation for this behaviour, according to sociobiological theory, is simply that as these monkeys have no investment in the genes of these infants, the sooner the infants are out of the way the more quickly the adults can produce offspring of their own. On the other hand, sociobiologists point to examples of non-genetic inspired altruism where infant birds and animals are nurtured and protected by non-relatives. Such behaviour is attributed to a species survival instinct and, it is argued, takes place only where there are benefits for the giver (Barash 1981: 132–69).

In a more recently reported study, Maestripieri *et al.* (1997) found evidence of intergenerational transmission of physical abuse of infant macaque monkeys in a longitudinal study covering 30 years.

The views of Krugman (1998) show how far thinking moved on in the 1990s in relation to genetics and child abuse. He described an experiment carried out in the USA comparing the nurturing behaviours of two mice, one of which had been deprived of a single gene:

> One mother mouse is in a cage with her newborn pups nursing avidly in a nest she made in the corner of the cage. The other mother is sitting (she even looks depressed) in the corner of her cage. There is no nest and all of her pups are dead at 24 hours of age.
>
> (Krugman 1998: 477)

Krugman asserted that these sorts of studies should be further explored:

> Some of us who've spent most of our time worrying about global issues find it pretty difficult to focus on single genes, but I would suggest that if we're going to get anywhere in this field, we need to start bringing neuroscientists, geneticists and others together with us, to just sit down and talk.
>
> (Krugman 1998: 478)

It is hard to know what weight to give to such ideas. While much of the theorizing of sociobiologists seems to be reductionist and over-stated, it does remind us of the part that instinct can play in certain behaviours and that it is a variable not to be overlooked or completely dismissed. Unthinking and indiscriminate use of such theory could, however, fuel prejudice and lead to over-reliance on common sense (and instinct!) as a tool for understanding the way in which people behave.

Attachment theory and child abuse

Attachment theory was described by Crittenden and Ainsworth (1989) as:

> a relatively new, open-ended theory with eclectic underpinnings. Intended as a revision of psychoanalytic theory, particularly Freudian instinct theory and metapsychology, it has been infused by present-day biological principles with an emphasis on ethology and evolutionary theory, as well as by control-systems theory and cognitive psychology.
>
> (Crittendon and Ainsworth 1989: 435)

The main theoretical tenets of attachment theory are derived from the work of one person, John Bowlby (1971). In the period immediately after the Second World War, he carried out studies into the nature and effects of maternal deprivation on young children (Bowlby 1951). He initially theorized that any significant separation of a child from the mother in the first five years of life could have deleterious effects on its emotional development and could lead to a variety of psychological and social difficulties in later life, such as the development of an affectionless personality and becoming a juvenile delinquent. Originally, the reasoning for this process was derived from psychodynamic theory, that is that the child developed a psychologically healthy sense of self through consistently rewarding contact with the mother. As his work developed, Bowlby drew more and more from the biological sciences and animal behaviour and placed more emphasis on the physical aspects of mother–child bonding and attachment. In the final outcome he argued that a child properly attached to the mother gains the dual benefit of physical protection and psychological security. He saw the process of attachment as an instinctive, genetically determined, two-way, symbiotic process.

Bowlby's early theorizing was criticized by Rutter (1978) for not taking into account the fact that the child could become attached to other significant figures as well as the mother. What was important, according to Rutter's argument, was the consistency and the positive nature of the relationship. Thus the roles of the father and other relatives in the emotional development of the child needed to be given more consideration.

Feminists have criticized attachment theory on the grounds that it has limiting and restrictive implications for women, because of its prescription that mothers should be in close proximity to their children for the whole of their infancy. Most attachment theorists now agree that children at around the age of 3 can cope with separation because they can by use of language and reasoning understand and accept explanations of what is happening.

Until the late 1980s, attachment theory was not directly applied to the problem of child abuse, though it has had a major influence on general child care policy and practice. Currently, poor attachment experiences are seen to be both a cause and a consequence of child abuse. Crittenden and Ainsworth (1989) argued that repeated consistent and rewarding interactions between a mother and child lead to high self-esteem and the capacity to trust. Non-responsive, rejecting and inconsistent responses from the mother lead to anxiety, insecurity, a lack of self-worth and an inability to relate to others. This problematic interaction is considered to lessen the child's chances of making satisfying peer relationships later on because a sense of self and trust of others, which are essential to this process, do not exist. The pattern may then be repeated with the child's own children, thus providing some explanation of how abuse is transmitted from one generation to the next (see Morton and Browne 1998). This process is not considered inevitable because the effects of poor early attachment experiences are thought to be remediable by attachment to a surrogate figure or by successful counselling.

Various studies of different kinds have been carried out to test attachment theory in relation to physical abuse and neglect (see Frodi and Lamb 1980; Egeland and Vaughan 1981; Main and Goldwyn 1984). All demonstrate connections between poor parent–child relationships and child abuse. Frodi and Lamb (1980), for instance, found that adults known to have abused children were both more aroused by children's crying and less responsive to their smiles than adults with no known record of abuse. Other studies (Gray *et al.* 1977; Browne and Saqi 1988) have produced evidence to support this connection between parental non-responsiveness and later abuse and neglect.

What are the strengths and weaknesses of this theoretical approach? The strengths lie in its convincing and detailed explanation of the process whereby abuse and neglect potential can be derived from poor adult–child relationships and be transmitted through them (see Argles 1980). The weaknesses lie, first, in the theory's failure to account more fully for the fact that the majority of parents who have been abused themselves do not go on to abuse their own children and, second, in the fact that insufficient account is taken of the total dynamics of the family: the focus is almost exclusively on the mother–child dyad. One could also argue that the theory does not take into account social stress factors, such as poverty and unemployment. However, Crittenden and Ainsworth (1989) did not totally ignore these factors. They acknowledged the high incidence of abuse among poor families and the impact of environmental stress, but pointed out that:

> Knowing the nature of family attachment relationships and the individuals' associated representational models should enable one to specify more precisely which families and/or individuals will be the most vulnerable to external stressors.
>
> (Crittenden and Ainsworth 1989: 458)

It should be noted that attachment theory has not been specifically used to explain sexual abuse of children, though (as noted in Chapter 7), it has been argued that where men are involved early on in the care of children there is reason to believe that such abuse is less likely to occur (Parker and Parker 1986).

Psychodynamic theory and physical child abuse and neglect

There is considerable overlap between psychodynamic theorizing about parent–child relationships and that of attachment theory and it is not easy to disentangle these two approaches. The main difference is that attachment theorists consider that these relationships are governed by instinct, whereas psychodynamic theory emphasizes the importance of internal mental processes in the way in which these relationships unfold.

Freud's work forms the kernel of psychodynamic thought, but it has been subjected to considerable variation by his followers. There are several good overviews of Freudian theory.[2] The key arguments of this perspective are that human beings mentally adapt their instinctive drives to the demands and requirements of their social circumstances. In the process of so doing, they develop personality traits that persist throughout life and influence their relationships with others. Freud's belief was that the dominant human instinctual drive was libidinal or sexual. He also theorized that very young children had such sexual drives and he devised an elaborate explanation of how these were moulded into pro-social behaviours and internalized to shape an individual's character.

Summarized very briefly, Freud postulated that in the first five years of life infants went through three psychosexual stages: the oral, the anal and the genital. These stages of development were linked to sources of physical pleasure – the oral stage to feeding, the anal stage to elimination and the genital stage to sexual stimulation. For Freud, socialization meant the suppression of these pleasures in order to function as a responsible person in society. Parents carried out this repressive/socializing task. As a result, childhood sexuality went through a latency stage only to reassert itself in adolescence, by which time individuals were considered to be more able to manage their libido for themselves. As a result of this process, the psyche of each individual was made up of the id (libidinal drive), the superego (the conscience or voice of the parent, which repressed the id) and the ego (the integrating element which balanced the id and superego and formed the visible or social aspect of the personality). The personality was also made up of different levels of consciousness as a result of this socializing process – the conscious (that part of the mind used in everyday life), the preconscious (that part of the mind from which past material could be summoned with prompting) and the unconscious (that part of the mind to which libidinal drives and urges had been exiled; these were normally unavailable to consciousness).

How does this relate to child abuse? With regard to physical abuse, Freudian or psychodynamic theory has been the most dominant explanatory model since its rediscovery in 1962. Yet this has rarely been made fully explicit. Sweet and Resick (1979) commented on this, pointing out that although most of the literature on child maltreatment has been influenced by psychodynamic concepts there have been few comprehensive attempts to construct a psychodynamic theory of child abuse. Steele and Pollock's (1974) account of child abuse causation is still probably the best example of a psychodynamic explanation. They considered that physical abuse was associated with a breakdown in motherliness. In terms of Freudian psychodynamics, Steele and Pollock (1974) hypothesized that from the very early stages the children of abusing parents are not responded to in a way that helps them to progress through all the necessary psychosexual stages. They are frustrated by lack of adequate response almost from the first contact and, therefore, are unlikely to develop the sort of integrated personality that enables them to relate responsively to others:

> Stimulation of the aggressive drive with its accompanying anger toward the frustrating caretaker, coupled with the parallel development of strict superego rudiments, inevitably leads to a strong sense of guilt. This guilt, largely unconscious, predominantly in relation to the mother, persists throughout the patient's life and leads to turning much of the aggression inward towards the self. When the parent misidentifies the infant as the embodiment of his own bad self, the full aggression of his punitive superego can be directed outward toward the child.
>
> (Steele and Pollock 1974: 122)

Thus, put simply, child abuse is seen to be the result of excessive superego demands.

The role of the non-abusing parent was not ignored by Steele and Pollock (1974), nor was the contribution that a child might make.[3] However, as in the case of attachment theory, the main focus is on the mother–child dyad. From the psychodynamic perspective, all other factors are secondary. The mother's psychological make-up (and occasionally the father's as well) is the key to the issue.

Psychological treatment, focusing on improving the parent's ability to relate to other people, is seen to be the solution to the problem. Such treatment is to be achieved by insight development (through a psychotherapist) and by the effects of a rewarding relationship with a social worker over a period of time. This model of response remained a major influence on both American and British child protection work up to the mid-1980s (see Letourneau 1981; Halston and Richards 1982).

The strengths of this approach, as with attachment theory, are that it can help professionals to understand the intrapersonal and interpersonal dynamics of child abuse and point to intervention aims and strategies. It is still hard for many in the child protection field to comprehend and tolerate violence to children; the psychodynamic approach provides a tool for this purpose. The weaknesses lie in the very heavy focus placed on women as the key carers without sufficient consideration of the circumstances in which they are operating and in the lack of attention to social and environmental factors.[4]

Psychodynamic theory and child sexual abuse

With regard to the sexual abuse of children, psychodynamic thought has rather a mixed history. According to Jeffrey Masson (1984), Freud, before his development of the psychosexual personality theories outlined above, hypothesized that hysteria in women may have been caused by their being sexually abused as children. This hypothesis was based on disclosures to him by women whom he was treating. He relayed his ideas to fellow doctors in Vienna, but they rejected his hypothesis mainly because, since hysteria was such a commonly diagnosed illness, the implication was that incestuous abuse was of epidemic proportions. Freud's response was to go away and look at his material again. Soon after, he laid the foundations of the theory of psychosexual development. Reference has already been made to the oral, anal and genital stages. With regard to the last, Freud hypothesized that, as part of their normal development, boys and girls at the genital stage 'desired' their parents of the opposite sex. This desire was repressed and the repression led to modelling along the lines of the same sex parent. When this process was disturbed, this led to developmental problems and the possibility of neurosis. Thus Freud argued that when he dealt with adults with such neuroses and tried to help them unlock these childhood repressions, it was not surprising that a lot of sexual material should arise. However, contrary to his original view, he saw these accounts as fantasies or wish-fulfilments rather than as recollections of fact.

Such theorizing was highly influential in psychoanalytic circles and was one factor in predisposing psychotherapists and psychiatrists for many years to disbelieve accounts of sexual abuse. Since the mid-1980s, as a result of increased general awareness of the problem, there is now a strong 'believing' school among psychoanalysts, the most famous example being Alice Miller (1985).

Psychoanalysts as a whole, however, have still not theorized about why child sexual abuse happens. Most would consider such abuse to have a very damaging effect on personality development, particularly if it took place in the first five years of a child's life, because of its distorting effect on the process of psychosexual development, but little has been written from this point of view about the causation of sexual abuse. Finkelhor et al. (1986), reviewing research on child sexual abusers, found two main views among psychoanalytic writing on this subject: first, that they have arrested psychosexual development and choose to relate at a child's emotional level; second, that they have general low self-esteem and, therefore, that they gain a sense of dominance and control by victimizing children. However, neither explanation properly explains why such people resort to sexual abuse in response to these emotional difficulties.

Learning theory and child abuse

Learning theory, while embracing many different approaches, is based on the deceptively simple view that behaviour is shaped, or learned, by the interaction of an individual with the environment. The internal processes described by psychoanalysts are completely rejected. Classical learning theorists (Pavlov 1927; Skinner 1953) see behaviour as a response conditioned by external stimuli or reinforcers and dismiss the notion of any internal functioning at all. From this point of view, what is not observable does not exist. However, since this early theorizing, learning theorists such as Bandura (1965) and Michenbaum (1977) have incorporated social modelling and the notion of internal cognitive reasoning processes into their analyses of how behaviour operates, and these more complex theories are generally accepted by most learning theorists now.

From this general perspective, child abuse is a problem resulting neither from personality traits nor from lack of attachment. Rather it is largely the result of having learned dysfunctional child care practices or, alternatively, of not having learned functional child care practices. The issue of punishment looms large here. Adults who have themselves experienced punitive treatment may well rely on such methods to discipline their own children. Most learning theorists see punishment as effective in the short term, but less so in the long term. It also has unwanted side-effects for both the punisher and the punished. The dysfunctional effects of punishment have been put forward as important reasons for banning all forms of corporal punishment (see Leach 1999). Positive reinforcement of pro-social behaviours and negative reinforcement (such as ignoring) of antisocial behaviours are seen as more effective and enduring influences on behaviour.

Dubanoski *et al.* (1978) described a set of behavioural explanations of why children are physically abused:

- parents may lack effective child management techniques
- parents may deliberately use punitive child-rearing practices
- the abuse may result from explosive acts triggered by the child
- there may be a high level of stress
- parents may have seriously negative attitudes towards the child.

Each of these problems might lead to the need for a variety of responses, including teaching new techniques, teaching self-control and focusing on attitude change.

Learning theorists have been applying their ideas to child abuse cases in the USA and Britain since the mid-1970s (see Isaacs 1982). In Britain, McAuley and McAuley (1977), Reavley and Gilbert (1979) and Smith and Rachman (1984) have all reported on interventions using learning theory approaches to modify parenting behaviours in families where physical abuse has occurred. The general finding has been that simply teaching new child management techniques is in many cases inadequate. There is need for attitudinal change on the part of parents as well, particularly where problems have been well established over a long period of time and motivation for change is low. Generally the results of behavioural interventions into child abuse have not been impressive. In the USA, there are more positive reports of behavioural interventions (see Crozier and Katz 1979; Denicola and Sandler 1980; Wolfe *et al.* 1981). The numbers in the samples are, however, small. Smith (1984) attributes the relative success of these interventions to the fact that therapeutic change is more embedded in US culture and that intervention programmes there are frequently enforced with the full backing of the courts.

The strengths of the learning theory perspective lie to some extent in its clarity and specificity. The learning theorist intervening in a case of child abuse would, for instance, focus on the actuality of the abuse, the situational factors, the antecedents and the consequences of the event, the attributions placed on the child by the parents, and their attitudes towards punishment and control. The personality of the parents and their developmental history would not be a major concern. There is also more potential for change than with the psychodynamic perspective, in that early experiences are not considered to be as deterministic.

Learning theory suffers from the same weaknesses as those of other psychological theories so far reviewed, namely that it often focuses on the individual abuser to the exclusion of the impact of wider networks. It may be that the strength of learning theory with regard to child abuse is also its weakness: it runs the risk of oversimplifying the problem in its search for clarity. In addition, it has so far paid little direct attention to the issue of child sexual abuse.

Cognitive approaches to child abuse

Cognitive approaches merge to a large extent with modern learning theory approaches. However, there is a growing interest, particularly in the USA (Newberger and White 1989), in the application of cognitive theory principles to the understanding of child abuse. The essential feature of this approach is that the way people perceive, order, construct and think about the world is an important key to their behaviour. In the previous section, it was noted that parental attitudes were perceived to be important, as well as their actual behaviour. Cognitive theorists point to the value of finding out how parents who have abused children perceive that child's behaviour. Larrance and Twentyman (1983) argue that attribution theory could help to explain why parents who have not been abused as children do abuse as adults.

Their argument is that they may have developed a 'frame' or view on a child and/or on themselves that leads on to child abuse.

Newberger and White (1989) put forward a useful model of levels of parental awareness. At the first level, the child is seen by the parents purely as an extension of themselves. At the second level, the parents ascribe conventional roles to the child. At the third level, the child is seen by the parents as an individual with its own changing needs. They argue that abuse is more likely to take place when parents are at the first level. Although most parents progress to the highest level with time and experience and without outside help or intervention, this is not true in all cases. According to this view, intervention must be focused on helping parents to perceive their children differently, and such activity can help to prevent recurrence of abuse.

There is not much information about the use of cognitive approaches in child protection practice. In Britain, Scott (1989) developed such work with general child care problems with some success, but, as with the behavioural approach, such success has been achieved with the less complex and less well-established problems.

Social psychological theories

In this section attention will be paid to theories that consider behaviour

- to be a product of interaction between individuals
- to be determined by family dynamics
- to be influenced by social networks and supports.

These approaches may be termed middle range in that they fall between focus on the individual and focus on broader social factors. Essentially the relationships between individuals and their immediate environments are seen as key determinants from these perspectives. The three areas of interaction have been separated from each other for analytic purposes, but many theorists of these persuasions see close linkages between them.

Individual interactionist perspectives and child abuse

The key defining factor of the individual interactionist approach is that behaviour is seen to be determined less by intrapersonal factors such as prior experiences, or by learning, and more by interactions between people. From this perspective, greater attention is placed on the dynamics of current relationships than on parental background or characteristics. Thus, interactionists take the child's contribution to situations of abuse much more into account, and also that of the spouse or partner (Kadushin and Martin 1981).

A climate of abuse can result from parents lacking skills to cope with difficult behaviour and from certain children continually exposing that inadequacy. From this perspective, the combination of factors is as important as the weight of them, if not more so. Thus, a difficult crying baby with two parents with low tolerance of stress and high aggression levels is particularly at risk, whereas a more easily comforted and responsive child with parents who have the same characteristics may not be. The child can, from this perspective, reward the parents and enhance their skills or further deskill them and lower their self-esteem. Similarly the parents' responses will affect the responses of the child in a circular process. Wolfe (1985) argued in similar vein to Larrance and Twentyman (1983) that parents do not have to have been abused themselves as children for them to abuse their own children. His explanation is different, however, in that he sees violence as a product of interactional events rather than of internal attribution processes. Wolfe (1985) argued that it is possible for a frame of violence to develop within families. Similarly, Dibble and Straus (1980) pointed out that violence to children can and does take place in families where parental attitudes are disapproving of such violence. This, they argued, is because such violence is often situational, not a product of attitudes. Their study involved only families with two parents and they found that violent behaviour on the part of one parent was likely to influence the other parent to be violent even if he or she was personally opposed to using violence against children. These studies lend support to the view that violence breeds violence.

This perspective on violence in the family offers another dimension with regard to the dynamics of why and how physical abuse of children occurs and persists. However, as is true of all the perspectives so far considered, a major weakness is that individuals are seen in isolation from wider social influences and stresses.

Family dysfunction theory and child abuse

Family dysfunction theory broadens the focus a little more in that its concern is with the impact of family dynamics on the behaviour of its members. This theory and family therapy, the treatment method derived from it, originated within the field of psychiatry and the aetiology of mental illness.

Family therapy is a theoretically eclectic discipline. Initially it drew mainly from psychodynamic theory and concentrated on the impact of family life on the psychological development of the individual. However, most current practitioners adopt a systems perspective based on the work of Minuchin (1974), which theorizes that there are two main subsystems within the family, that of the parents and that of children, and emphasizes the need for boundaries (with some degree of permeability) to be maintained between the two in order to ensure a healthy climate for all family members. Therapy is focused on examining the nature of current boundaries and on improving communication between family members. Another family therapy approach is termed 'strategic'. Family therapists of this school see the family as a powerful system that resists attempts to change it from the outside (Dale *et al.* 1983). Carefully worked out tactics and strategies are needed to break down this resistance to create the best conditions for change.

With regard to physical child abuse, dysfunctional family theory has not had widespread influence as an explanatory theory. However, family therapy techniques as a mode of intervention have more recently attracted attention. Asen *et al.* (1989) focused on how family dynamics contribute to abuse. They referred to the notion of stand-in abuse where the child is subjected to violence by its parent as a means of 'getting at' the other parent. The notion of a child as 'scapegoat', the bad one in the family and the reason for all the family's ills, is another example of a family dysfunction explanation of child mistreatment. Reder *et al.* (1993) used material from public inquiry reports to examine both intrafamilial dynamics and professional–parent dynamics in cases where children are seriously abused or killed. They focused particularly on the way in which parents tend to oscillate between revealing what is going on (what are termed covert warnings) and concealing it. There is a general lack of focus on causes of behaviour among family therapists. Their concern is with the here-and-now dynamics of family life and how to break or change patterns of behaviour. From this point of view, the notion of 'cause' in the linear cause-and-effect sense is seen to be less relevant than the process.

Family therapy and child sexual abuse

In contrast to its limited impact on the physical abuse field in Britain, family therapy thinking has played a major role in the explanation of the cause of child sexual abuse. This is largely due to the pioneering work of Ben-Tovim *et al.* (1988) at the Great Ormond Street Hospital referred to in Chapter 3. Their approach, which incorporates both psychodynamic and systems theories, is broadly based on the hypothesis that child sexual abuse serves the function of keeping together families that would otherwise collapse. The classic scenario is that of the abuse of a teenage daughter by her father, who is considered to be seeking emotional and sexual gratification because communication and sexual relations with his wife have broken down. It is believed in many cases that the wife/mother knows (whether consciously or subconsciously is not made clear) what is happening and passively colludes in the continuance of this situation. This collusion is thought to serve the function of freeing her from responsibility without sacrificing the unity of the family. The solution to the problem is seen to be one of opening up the secret to all family members, disentangling the knotted relationships and freeing individuals to decide on their futures. The means for achieving this is by family meetings and the use of family therapy techniques.

The strengths of the family dysfunction approach are that it heightens awareness of the powerful nexus of relationships that the family can be sheltering and demonstrates how it can sustain unacceptable forms of abuse. However, it suffers from the problem of many systems-based theories in that although it describes well how dysfunctional families operate, it is much more limited in explaining the reason why they function in the way that they do. The Great Ormond Street team explained sexual abuse by reference to the emotional need of the perpetrator and the structural dependence on adults of the child victim. Feminist critiques of family dysfunction theory have stressed the lack of attention paid to gender power relations (see pp. 150–1). Family therapy thinking has also been criticized for focusing too much on the family as a closed system cut off from wider systems and social influences. There is evidence of the development of more flexible family dysfunction approaches that take into account both these issues (Treacher and Carpenter 1984; Barratt *et al.* 1990; Masson and O'Byrne 1990; Jenkins and Asen 1992). A final criticism is that the explanatory value of the family dysfunction approach is limited to the types of abuse situations outlined above. It does not help to explain the wide range of forms of sexual abuse that can take place in families, such as abuse of infants and abuse by siblings (see Corby 1998).

Social ecological approaches

General systems theory has been adapted by social work theorists in the USA and Britain to broaden traditional emphasis on personal problems and to move away from concentration on personal pathology (Pincus and Minahan 1973). The influence of systems theory in understanding and interpreting social problems has been particularly influential in the USA with the development of general concerns about the environment. Germain and Gitterman (1980) provided a good example of the thinking behind this model:

The ecological perspective provides an adaptive, evolutionary view of human beings in constant interchange with all elements of their environment. Human beings change their physical and social environments and are changed by them through a process of continuous reciprocal adaptation . . . Like all living systems,

human beings must maintain a goodness-of-fit with the environment. The Darwinian concept of 'fit' applies both to organisms
and their environments: to the fitness of the environment and
the fitness of the organism, each with the other and through
which both prosper.

(Germain and Gitterman 1980: 5–6)

Such thinking has not been directly and specifically applied to child
abuse in Britain except in a general way with regard to social isolation. In the USA, however, direct attention has been paid to the
way in which the interrelationship between human beings and their
social environment can have an impact on the incidence of child
maltreatment.

From this perspective, human behaviour is more influenced, or
determined, by the context in which a person lives rather than purely
by intrapersonal or interpersonal factors. In the particular case of
child abuse, it is hypothesized that where environmental conditions
are unfavourable to families, the incidence of abuse is likely to be
higher. In the USA, Garbarino (1977, 1982) has been particularly
active in exploring these connections. He found in both rural and
urban areas that officially reported abuse was higher in those neighbourhoods where indicators of social stress, population mobility and poverty were highest. A major factor was seen to be isolation from possible
support systems, be they the extended family or community-based
systems such as neighbourhood centres and day-care facilities: 'A strong
pro-social neighbourhood climate can have a beneficial impact – by
increasing participation – on persons whose individual predilection is
to be isolated' (Garbarino and Crouter 1978: 606).

Garbarino (1977) links this theoretical approach to others in that he
does not preclude individual history as an additional causative factor
and he acknowledges that culture plays a part, in that, if there were
not cultural justification for the use of force against children (see
pp. 147–8), then it would not happen, however deprived the conditions in which families were living (Garbarino 1977). Nevertheless,
given these factors, stress, created from living in environments that
are not conducive to psychological health and development, is seen
to be a major contributory factor to child mistreatment and points to
solutions other than focus on the individual, most notably community-
based initiatives to break down isolation and to create a sense of
belonging and shared problems. In Britain, examples of this type of
approach are to be found in Holman (1988), but in general initiatives
around the needs of communities as a whole have declined since the
1970s. Child protection work has 'opened up' to some degree with
greater use of family centres (see Chapter 10), but the model of treatment used in such centres tends to operate at the individual and
familial level.

There are difficulties with 'proving' the validity of this theory, not least because of the fact that poorer communities are more likely to come under the close surveillance of public authorities and, therefore, produce higher official rates of abuse. There is also a need for closer attention to be paid to which particular deficits in what circumstances contribute to child maltreatment and the process by which this happens (see Seagull 1987; Coohey 1996). Cohen and Adler (1986), looking more broadly at social network interventions, are opposed to the use of community-based initiatives as the solution to all social problems. They are concerned that they could be used as cheap-option cure-alls, mirroring the current debate in Britain about community care packages for mentally ill and elderly people.

The main strength of the social ecological approach lies in the way in which it broadens the scope of thinking about why abuse of children occurs. It shifts the focus from individual pathology to the influence of the immediate environment and the need to tackle the problem at that level. At the same time many exponents of this approach pay little attention to political factors that contribute to the deterioration of neighbourhoods and the disorganization and break-up of social networks. Attention to these issues might well lead to quite different solutions to the problem.

Sociological perspectives

Sociological perspectives on child abuse did not have a major influence on child protection thinking and work in Britain before the 1990s, except in the case of sexual abuse and gender issues. The reason for this is twofold. First, such perspectives do not provide clear indicators for practice in that they look broadly at the conditions which create the climate for child abuse rather than at how this works out in individual cases (Corby 1991). Second, many sociological perspectives provide a challenge to those who are intervening into families to protect children, in that they question the ethics and politics of mainstream assumptions (Howe 1991). Thus, they have an unsettling quality in that they locate the 'cause' of the problem outside the sphere of influence of the professional worker and they consequently pose uncomfortable questions about the validity of that professional intervention. To some degree, Department of Health initiatives in the second half of the 1990s (see Chapter 4) have attempted to redress the balance in that they have paid greater attention to stress as a causative factor in certain types of child abuse and to the need for broader-based assessments of families referred for child protection concerns.

The main sociological perspectives to be considered in this section are those that have been articulated by researchers and others involved in the child abuse field:

- the social cultural perspective, which points to linkages between child abuse and general social approval of the use of violence to maintain control and order
- the social structural perspective, which relates child abuse to the maintenance of general inequality in northern industrialized societies
- perspectives that link child abuse to gender and generational inequality, that is feminist and children's rights perspectives.

The social cultural perspective and child abuse

The work of Straus and Gelles (1986) in the USA has already been referred to several times in relation to their national surveys into the incidence of physical child abuse (see Chapter 5). In these studies, they and their colleagues reported high levels of intrafamilial violence of all kinds. They came to the conclusion that such violence was the norm and that individuals were more likely to be subjected to violent acts within families than outside them. In an attempt to explain these high rates, they argued that violence is a socially sanctioned general form of maintaining order and that it is approved of as a form of child control by most people in US society. It can be argued from this perspective that a society that approves of the corporal punishment of children in schools and endorses the old adage 'spare the rod and spoil the child' sets the scene for a variety of unwanted forms of violence, of which physical child abuse is one. Thus, child abuse is seen to be on the same spectrum as socially approved forms of violence rather than as a separate pathological phenomenon.

Goode (1971) examines the process whereby such culturally approved violence takes hold. The family is seen as a power system mirroring that of the wider society (see also Wolff 1981). Conformity and compliance with rules are seen as desirable and are ultimately enforced by the use of violence (or the threat of it). Both children and parents are socialized into believing that this type of rule enforcement is legitimate and ultimately beneficial. Goode (1971) goes on to explain why he believes that use of violent force is more common among poorer families. Parents with more resources at their disposal are less likely to resort to overt use of force. Normally they will be able to maintain control by other means. Poorer parents with less resources have fewer alternatives to violence for asserting their wills.

Gelles and Cornell (1985) argued that an important contributory factor to child and other forms of intrafamilial abuse is the likelihood that the perpetrator will get away with it, partly because it takes place within the confines of the family and is, therefore, difficult to prove in the world outside (that is in a court of law) and partly because of the state's traditional reluctance to interfere in family affairs.

Straus (1994) pointed to the dysfunctions of corporal punishment for individuals in later life (which can include lowered self-esteem and poor social relationship skills), their families (as a result of the inter-generational transmission of punitive parenting) and for society as a whole which is increasingly looking in the job market for individuals with flexible problem-solving skills, a style of behaviour not generally created by the use of physical punishment as a key form of discipline.

From this perspective, it is clear that there is a need for change at a broad societal level to the way in which we treat and control children. There is a need to encourage non-violent means of ensuring pro-social behaviour. As we saw in Chapter 4, there have been moves in this direction in Britain since 1998. However, other European countries have been much more proactive in this respect; in Sweden where the ban on use of physical punishment of children by parents has been in operation the longest, there has been some degree of success in terms of rates of reported child abuse (Gelles and Edfeldt 1986).

The same sort of analysis can be applied to sexual abuse: that because sexual exploitation of women and, to a lesser extent, of children, is societally tolerated in, for instance, art, cinema, advertising and pros-titution, a climate is set whereby sexual abuse results. Again, from this perspective, it is seen as part of a continuum rather than as an act of a totally different quality or dimension.

The strengths of the social cultural perspective are that they broaden the focus in comparison with psychological and social psychological theories and help in the understanding of how societal influences can contribute to the incidence and form of child mistreatment despite the fact that society officially sets out to reduce and prevent such occurrences. The implications for social policy are that there is a need to tackle the issue on a broader front and that intervention into individual cases alone is not sufficient for dealing with the problem. The major weakness of this perspective lies in the fact that it does not help to explain why some people within our flawed culture abuse and others do not.

The social structural perspective and child abuse

Gil's research and writing, already frequently referred to, form the cornerstone of this perspective. Gil's (1970) early work convinced him that child abuse was class-related and that 'psychological' explanations of abuse by themselves were too narrow and grossly underestimated the contribution of stress, caused by poverty and material deprivation, to the causation of child abuse.

He developed his ideas further to lay some of the blame for child abuse on the policies of the state (Gil 1975, 1978). He put forward a broad definition of abuse (see Chapter 4), which included all children whose developmental needs could not be met, whatever the reason. This definition clearly places responsibility for child abuse on the state over and above the person who actually abuses, on the grounds that it sanctions inequality and low standards of housing, health, education and leisure for the children of the poor. From this point of view, the state, far from being the benign rescuer of children when parents ill-treat them, is actually the villain of the piece because it abuses children directly by its failure to provide adequate facilities for them to lead a fulfilling life, and it also creates stresses for parents that increase the likelihood of their committing acts of abuse or neglect. Parton (1985) has lent support to this perspective in Britain:

> Child abuse is strongly related to class, inequality and poverty both in terms of prevalence and severity . . . Locating the problem in terms of social structural factors has important implications for the way we define the problem, the way we explain it and the best way of doing something about it. For solving the problem requires a realignment in social policy which recognises the necessity of attacking the social, economic and cultural conditions associated with the abuse.
>
> (Parton 1985: 175–6)

The strength of the social structural approach is that it does justice to the accepted fact that physical child abuse has a close association with deprivation. As we have seen, this is particularly so with regard to neglect (see Wolock and Horowitz 1984). Its weakness lies in the fact that not all poor people abuse their children and, therefore, it is not a sufficient explanation. This perspective has so far not taken into account structural factors other than class and poverty. In particular it has been silent on the issue of gender and generational inequalities (Parton 1990). Finally, it does not address the issue of the aetiology of child sexual abuse, which is generally considered not to be linked to class and poverty.

The social structural approach has not had a great deal of support in child abuse circles. Pelton (1978) pointed to the fact that structural inequality explanations pose a threat to those who espouse clinical and medical approaches to child abuse. Other writers have seen Gil's views as 'idealistic' (Greenland 1987) or beyond the scope of the helping professions and, therefore, not applicable to day-to-day practice. As noted in Chapter 4, current child protection policy in Britain is beginning to take into account structural inequality or social exclusion, as it is currently termed, in the understanding and assessment of child protection referrals. However (as noted earlier), there is some concern that the resources required to meet some of the needs uncovered by these broader assessments cannot be met by local government expenditure (see Tunstill 1997). There is need for a much more concerted national effort to tackle the forms of exclusion and disadvantage that, according to social structural theorization, are causative factors behind child abuse.

The feminist perspective and child abuse

Most of the perspectives so far outlined are considered by feminist thinkers to be gender-blind. All of the psychological perspectives assume that women are the key carers of children and that, if things go wrong, then the focus must fall on their behaviour. The interactionist perspectives broaden the focus, but assume an equal power base between men and women. Neither of the two sociological perspectives discussed above pays much attention to the issue of gender.

A radical feminist perspective on the issue of child abuse began to emerge in the 1980s. The stimulus for this came from the 'discovery' of child sexual abuse, an act committed predominantly by males, and feminist explanations have been highly relevant to it. From this starting-point, the feminist perspective has now been applied to all forms of abuse.

The feminist perspective on child sexual abuse has been articulated by several writers in the USA and Britain (Rush 1980; Herman 1981; Dominelli 1986; Nelson 1987; Macleod and Saraga 1988; Driver and Droisen 1989). There is little equivocation about the reason for the existence of child sexual abuse and the form that it takes:

> Generally boys and men learn to experience their sexuality as an overwhelming and uncontrollable force; they learn to focus their sexual feelings on submissive objects, and they learn the assertion of their sexual desires, the expectation of having them serviced.
> (Macleod and Saraga 1988: 41)

Abuse in the form of violence against women is a normal feature of patriarchal relations. It is a major vehicle that men use in controlling women. As such it is the norm not an aberration. The widespread incidence of child sexual abuse reveals the extent to which men are prepared to wield sexual violence as a major weapon in asserting their authority over women (Dominelli 1986: 12).

The attention of these writers is not on individual males. Individual pathology is discounted as a cause of child abuse (as is family pathology). Rather, abuse is seen as an extreme example of institutionalized male power over females. The implications for policy of this perspective are similar in kind, if not focus, to those of the other sociological perspectives. Sexual abuse is an issue that needs tackling at a societal level as well as at the individual level. Men abuse children because of the general power imbalance between the sexes and the different forms of socialization that they experience as a result, not because of psychiatric illness or emotional deficits.

With regard to physical abuse and neglect, the issues for the feminist perspective are less clear-cut. As we have seen, women are as implicated in the physical abuse and neglect of children as well as men. Thus the argument that such abuse is created by the conditions of patriarchy does not sit as easily in this case as in that of sexual abuse. However (as argued in Chapter 7), women spend far more time with children than do men and cope with the stresses of child care, often with little support. The argument is taken further by some feminists in that they see the notion of motherhood, a product of patriarchy, which reinforces the idea that children's welfare and needs are best met by mothers, exacerbating the already existing stresses placed on women looking after children. Under such conditions, it is surprising that the numbers of women who abuse and neglect children do not vastly exceed those of men, and, from this point of view, men are disproportionately violent to children. The implication is that women's violence to children is much more likely to be stress-related than that of men. As we have already seen in Chapter 7, another area opened up by the feminist perspective is that of partner violence (Dobash and Dobash 1992) and its linkage with child abuse (Mullender and Morley 1994).

From this feminist perspective, the patriarchal nature of our society does, therefore, have a major role to play in the causation of physical abuse and neglect of children.

The strength of the feminist perspective on child abuse as a whole is that it opened up a dimension that recently has been missing from explanations about why child abuse occurs. Reference was made in Chapter 7 to the way in which (in the case of physical abuse and neglect) men seem to have been overlooked in terms of intervention. The feminist perspective points to the error in this in that understanding and challenging the nature of male–female power relations, at an institutional and individual level, is of major importance in the theory and practice of child protection work (see O'Hagan and Dillenberger 1995). The challenge should be both to the impositions placed on women within the family and to the way in which males are socialized (Hearn 1990). The weakness of the feminist perspective is that there is a danger that it can be used in a reductionist and exclusive way, attributing every ill to patriarchy and overriding all other explanatory accounts (see Featherstone and Lancaster 1997).

The children's rights perspective and child abuse

Freeman (1983) identified two main schools of thought on children's rights, the protectionist and the liberationist.

Protectionist thinking about children has been applied to child care issues through legislation since the late nineteenth century (see Chapter 3) and still underlies much of current policy and practice in the field of child abuse. Essentially the argument from this viewpoint is that children have the right to protection from their parents by outside bodies in circumstances where their health and welfare are at risk. In the absence of these conditions, parents have the responsibility of determining their children's rights up to prescribed ages.

The liberationist perspective is a product of the late 1960s and derives mainly from the field of education. Holt (1974) provided a good example of the extreme end of this type of thinking. His argument is that childhood is an oppressed status and that the current state of affairs in which parents grant concessions to children who have little redress against their actions and decisions is unjust and reinforces their oppression. He proposes a series of rights that children should have, such as the right to choose where to live, the right to vote and the right to have the same financial status as adults. In short, his view is that children should have exactly the same rights as adults. Age is seen as irrelevant and self-determination as paramount. Scarre (1980) pointed out some of the obvious weaknesses in this approach, most notably that children are both physically and emotionally dependent on their parents for several years. Paternalism is, from his viewpoint, a largely beneficial protective mechanism for children until they can reach maturity.

In the late 1980s and 1990s there was a shift in official thinking about children's rights away from a traditional protectionist perspective towards viewing children in a more independent light. This was largely due to events in Cleveland. The traditional view that children are either the responsibility of the family or, where abuse occurs, that of the state has been thrown into question by what happened there. The Cleveland report (Butler-Sloss 1988) was highly critical of the way in which children were treated during investigations. It pointed out that 'There is a danger that in looking to the welfare of children believed to be the victims of sexual abuse the children themselves may be overlooked. The child is a person not an object of concern' (Butler-Sloss 1988: 245). The 1989 Children Act also takes children's rights of this kind more closely into consideration.[5] However, neither the Cleveland report nor the 1989 Children Act could possibly be seen as liberationist in the way in which Holt (1974) proposed. In fact they reflect a half-way house position between the protectionist and liberationist viewpoints. Children's views are to be taken into account, but there is no suggestion that they should prevail.

In respect of physical abuse, the development of anti-corporal punishment legislation and policy reflects the influence of liberationist views. The thinking is clear: if children had the same rights in society as adults and, therefore, similar individual status (one that was not prescribed by family relations), they would be less likely to be the object of physical abuse and neglect. For instance, we do not consider it proper to smack adults for misbehaving. Were children to have individual rights without reference to their parents, we would not consider such treatment to be acceptable in their case either.

The main strength of the children's rights perspective is that it compels us to consider matters from the child's point of view as an individual rather than purely as a family member and points to changes in the status of children at a societal level as a solution to the widespread problem of child abuse. While the importance of this perspective has no bounds, it should be stressed that the notion of children's rights has a particular role to play in the protection of children living away from home. The various reports (see Chapter 4) on the care of children being looked after in local authority care and elsewhere demonstrate the consequences of children not being able to assert rights of complaint against those in power over them. Although there have been considerable general developments in the 1990s to establish and assert these rights – for instance, the UN Convention on the Rights of the Child, adopted by the United Nations in 1989 and ratified by the UK government in 1991, and the setting up of a formal representations procedure in the 1989 Children Act, there has not been any obvious evidence of improvement in this respect (see Lyon 1997).

The weakness of the children's rights perspective lies in the fact that most children living at home cannot be easily seen in isolation from their parents because of their dependence on them. Children's rights protagonists tend to ignore this fact and also the fact that many parents do not have the means to achieve the high standards that the children's rights perspective properly demands.

Concluding comments

Virtually all researchers into the field of child abuse point to the dangers of adopting single-cause explanations of the phenomenon. While some explanations may seem to be particularly useful for the understanding of certain forms of abuse (for example attachment theory appears to have particular relevance in the case of physical abuse or emotional rejection of young babies), they are unlikely to be sufficient in themselves.

There has been (and still is) a polarization between different perspectives on why child abuse occurs, with single explanations dominating in different camps. The most obvious example is the clash between the feminist perspective and that of family therapists over the aetiology of child sexual abuse. In the field of physical abuse, the case of Jasmine Beckford highlights the clash between psychological and sociological perspectives. The social workers in this case focused on improving the social circumstances of the parents of Jasmine by helping them find more suitable accommodation, by providing Jasmine's mother with supportive help at home and by obtaining nursery school provision for Jasmine. The focus was on external factors improving the quality of life, thereby reducing stress and enhancing parent–child relationships. The report criticized the social workers on a variety of grounds, including not taking into account the psychological background of the parents. With the value of hindsight, this criticism was justified and greater attention to interpersonal and intrapersonal factors may have led to greater caution in decision-making.

It is clear that social workers and other professional workers in this field need to be open to a wide range of explanations of child abuse in order to intervene effectively into families where children are thought to be at risk, even though this approach may be more complex than that of following a single theory. Attempts to integrate the different approaches to child abuse are being made. Belsky (1980), using an ecological framework, pointed to a four-level approach, that is ontogenic development, the microsystem, the exosystem and the macrosystem:

• ontogenic development is concerned with what the individual parents bring to the situation, their developmental background and experiences
• the microsystem is concerned with the interaction of individuals within the family
• the exosystem is concerned with the immediate social environment within which the family functions
• the macrosystem takes into account broader structural factors, such as cultural attitudes to violence.

The way in which these different systems interact is the key to the likelihood of abuse occurring or not (see also Ostbloom and Crase 1980; Wiehe 1989; Coohey and Braun 1997). All these integrative models have been devised with physical abuse in mind. Finkelhor *et al.* (1986) provided a similar type of model for child sexual abuse.

The way forward is clearly in the direction of further attempts at integrating ongoing research into the aetiology of child abuse. While practitioners may be more concerned with what is directly relevant to practice, it should be borne in mind that a broad range of integrated knowledge provides a strong base from which to operate. As Gordon (1989) persuasively argued, on the basis of her historical research into child protection agency records:

The most helpful social workers were those who understood family-violence problems to be simultaneously social structural and

personal in origin, and who therefore offered help in both dimen-
sions. Good caseworkers might help a family get relief, or medical
care, or a better apartment, and build a woman's or a child's self-
esteem by legitimating their claims and aspirations.

(Gordon 1989: 298)

Integrated thinking about the causation of child abuse does of course
have implications for far many others than front-line child protection workers. However much we develop understandings of abuse and
neglect at the microlevel, the implications of the broader sociological
theories of child abuse causation cannot be avoided by society as a
whole. They are that a more concerted effort needs to be made to give
consideration to child abuse prevention in all areas of planning and
policing of society.

Recommended reading

Belsky, J. (1980) Child maltreatment: an ecological integration, *American Psychologist*, 35: 320–35.
Jenkins, H. and Asen, K. (1992) Family therapy without the family: a framework for systemic practice, *Journal of Family Therapy*, 14: 1–14.
Mullender, A. and Morley, R. (1994) *Children Living with Domestic Violence:
Putting Men's Abuse of Women on the Child Care Agenda*. London: Whiting
and Birch.
Newberger, C. and White, K. (1989) Cognitive foundations for parental care,
in D. Cicchetti and V. Carlson (eds) *Child Maltreatment: Theory and Research
on the Causes and Consequences of Child Abuse and Neglect*. Cambridge: Cambridge University Press.
Parton, N. (1985) *The Politics of Child Abuse*. London: Macmillan.
Steele, B. and Pollock, C. (1974) A psychiatric study of parents who abuse
infants and small children, in R. Helfer and C. Kempe (eds) *The Battered
Child*, 2nd edn. Chicago: University of Chicago Press.

chapter **nine**

THE CONSEQUENCES OF CHILD ABUSE

Introduction

In the past there has been less attention paid to the consequences or effects on a child of being abused than to ways of preventing such abuse happening in the first place. This could not be so easily argued now. Particularly since the rediscovery of child sexual abuse in the 1980s, there has been an explosion of interest in, and studies of, the consequences both of this form of abuse and of all others as well. This concern with the effects of sexual abuse is largely attributable to the pressure of the feminist movement, but it may also reflect increasing societal concerns about risk to individuals identified by Beck (1992). He argued that such concerns are characteristic of modern, more affluent societies which possess increasingly more effective technological means of controlling large aspects of life and which thereby create a strong desire to reduce risk to a minimum. This argument has been applied to child abuse concerns generally (see Parton *et al.* 1996). However, it seems particularly persuasive in explaining the growth of attention paid to the consequences of abuse, because, as pointed out in Chapter 8 in relation to physical punishment of children, it is not only those who are abused who may pay a cost, but their relatives and society as well.

Moving on to the concerns of child protection policy-makers and practitioners, there are several good reasons for careful study of the consequences of child abuse. First, while there is no doubt that all abuse of children is likely to have harmful consequences, some forms of abuse may be more harmful than others and have different implications for intervention. There is the constant concern, stemming in Britain from events like those that took place in Cleveland and the Orkneys, that some forms of intervention may add to the harm already created by the abuse that the child has suffered rather than alleviate it. Knowing about the consequences of different forms and levels of abuse can make a key contribution to decisions about the best way to respond to it.

Second, there is a preventive aspect to focusing on the consequences of abuse. The issue of intergenerational transmission of abuse was discussed in Chapter 7. Greater focus on the effects of abuse can lead to better treatment measures, which may reduce the likelihood of abuse being repeated in the next generation.

Third, there is the issue of abuse survival. As we shall see later, there are children who, despite experiencing forms and degrees of abuse that would lead us to expect that they would be severely damaged as a result, appear to cope well and without apparent psychological ill-effects. Studying how these children successfully survive also has implications for intervention and treatment.

Research into the effects of child abuse suffers from similar problems and limitations to research considered in previous chapters. First, there are the same methodological issues with regard to sampling and the use of controls. Some studies use small clinical samples while others select their samples from a broader range of cases. Some studies do not use controls and those that do go to different lengths to match them with their samples. Second, there are the same problems about agreed definitions of what constitutes abuse. Lack of definitional clarity makes comparability between different studies difficult; it is not always possible to be sure that you are comparing like with like. Some studies are careful to differentiate between types of abuse and degrees of severity, while others are not.

In addition there are some problems that are particular to research into the consequences of abuse. These are, first, the difficulty of deciding on the length of time to be allowed for follow-up of cases and, second, the difficulty of establishing causal connections between abuse events and later behaviour. These problems are closely linked. Research that is carried out soon after the abuse has occurred will obviously miss out on evaluating longer-term effects. On the other hand, the greater the gap between the abuse event and the later behaviour, the less chance there is of causally linking the two because of the existence of more intervening variables. The following example demonstrates some of these issues.

The case of child sexual abuse and prostitution

Prostitution has been seen to be a consequence of sexual abuse. Silbert and Pines (1981) interviewed 200 juvenile and adult prostitutes in San Francisco. They found that 60 per cent had been sexually abused as children. On the face of it, this seems to provide reasonable proof that there is a direct connection between being sexually abused as a child and becoming a prostitute. However, as far as we know, the vast majority of sexually abused female children do not become prostitutes and, therefore, this uncritical reading of these findings is not acceptable. More information is needed to find out in more detail why and in what circumstances the abused women in this study turned to prostitution. Silbert and Pines (1981) did provide more details about the type of sexual abuse experienced by their sample: 60 per cent were abused by an average of two people over a period of 20 months; 66 per cent of these were abused by father figures and 82 per cent said that their abuse had been accompanied by some degree of force. Thus, these variables – length of time of abuse, the close relationship between abuser and abused and the use of violence or threats of violence – could be linked with the outcome of prostitution. However, despite this attempt to be more specific, the account is still deficient. There are many social, cultural, economic and interpersonal factors that may also have been important determinants of the later behaviour of these women, in addition to the fact that they were victims of serious sexual assault early in their lives. The latter may have a predisposing effect, but to reach the conclusion that prostitution is a direct consequence of sexual abuse is simplistic and misleading.

Most studies of the consequences of child abuse differentiate between short-term and long-term effects. In what follows, focus will be placed on the short- and long-term consequences of, first, physical abuse and neglect, with some reference to the impact of emotional abuse, and then on those relating to sexual abuse.

The consequences of physical abuse and neglect

Short- and medium-term effects on emotional development

Calam and Franchi (1987) provided a good overview of psychological characteristics displayed in the short term by children who are physically abused or neglected. Many of these characteristics can be seen as

survival tactics adopted by the powerless in the face of harsh or neglectful treatment. Such abused children develop a form of pseudo-
maturity that manifests itself in behaviour aimed at keeping their
parents happy. Generally they have a lack of appetite for, or confidence in, play. Such children become self-critical and lacking in
self-esteem. 'Frozen watchfulness' is another response, usually to more
extreme forms of deprivation, that is the child seems to be wary of
human contact and to lack emotional reaction. Hyperactivity and
inability to settle for any substantial length of time have also been
seen as typical of the behaviour of physically abused children. These
initial responses may or may not persist. Calam and Franchi (1987)
studied a small number of abused/neglected children attending an
NSPCC day centre with their mothers and came to the conclusion
that 'severity of injury was not the major determinant of the degree of
disturbances that they showed; the family environment that they
were continuing to experience was likely to play a more significant
part' (Calam and Franchi 1987: 191). From this viewpoint, this early
negative psychological development is caused not so much by the
actual physical abuse as by the way in which parents relate emotionally to their children, and it is maintained by the way in which they
continue to interact with them regardless of whether they use physical violence again or not.

Steele (1986), arguing along similar lines, stressed that the main
feature of being an abused child is inconsistent care, which in general
terms leads to a sense of insecurity. This evidences itself in low self-
esteem, problems in developing a sense of self-identity, a diminution
in the ability to cope with life and its stresses, a lack of ability to take
pleasure in things and to make lasting attachments, depression, delinquency and masochism. For Steele (1986), as for Calam and Franchi
(1987), physical abuse *per se* is not the issue. It is the emotional
quality of parenting that is the key:

> Physical abuse does not necessarily cause trouble. Most people
> have had physical injuries, fractures or bumps during childhood
> due to purely accidental causes and they have not been harmed
> by it because they have been comforted and cared for by good
> caregivers at the time of the incident. Damage comes when the
> injuries are inflicted by those to whom one looks for love and
> protection and there is no relief from the trauma.
>
> (Steele 1986: 283–4)

For Steele, the emotionally incapacitating effects of this type of
early mistreatment can be alleviated only by positive interpersonal
experiences.

Many researchers have found a correlation between physical abuse
and negative emotional consequences without being specific about

the dynamics of the process. Kinard (1980) reviewed nine studies carried out between 1971 and 1978 and found that, although the samples were small in size and were methodologically different, 'these investigations are remarkably consistent in the findings that abused children show substantial deficits in emotional development' (Kinard 1980: 452). He commented further: 'The results corroborate reports of case histories depicting the abused child as having a negative self-concept' (1980: 452). Toro (1982), Lamphear (1985) and Augoustinos (1987) carried out similar reviews of studies and Kinard's (1980) conclusions are largely confirmed.

Erickson *et al.* (1989) carried out a series of studies to discover the effects of different types of abuse on children. They studied four 'abused' groups of children over the first six years of their lives. These groups consisted of

- children who were physically abused
- children whose parents were hostile and verbally abusive
- children who were neglected
- children whose parents were psychologically unavailable (that is they were emotionally abusive).

Overall there were 84 'abused' children and they were compared with a control group of 85 'non-abused' children from similar socio-economic backgrounds. Children from all the 'abused' groups were generally rated as having less confidence and lower self-esteem than those in the control group. Differences between the groups, while not as clear-cut as in the comparison between abused and non-abused, were nevertheless apparent. At age 4, the neglected and emotionally abused children were the cause of most concern. With regard to the latter, the researchers write:

> The sharp decline in the intellectual functioning of these children, in their attachment disturbances and subsequent lack of social/emotional competence in a variety of situations is cause for great concern. The consequences of this form of maltreatment are particularly disturbing when considered in light of the fact that it is probably the least likely pattern of maltreatment to be detected.
>
> (Erickson *et al.* 1989: 667)

However, at age 6 these children, whose parents were described as psychologically unavailable, fared as well as the other groups of abused children. The group giving most cause for concern at this stage was the neglected children, who were very low achievers in school. Other studies have also pointed to the fact that neglected children seem to be lower in self-esteem than children who have been physically abused (Oates *et al.* 1985).

In Britain, the main study in this field is that of Lynch and Roberts (1982). They followed up 39 physically abused children four years after investigation and treatment. They compared the progress of these children with a similar number of their non-abused siblings. Their findings were in line with the US studies referred to so far, namely that generally the abused group were developmentally, emotionally, educationally and socially below the norms for children of their age. This was regardless of whether they had been removed from home or whether they remained with their parents receiving supportive help from outside agencies. With regard to psychological development only, these abused children were commonly described as showing signs of anxiety, extreme shyness and fear of failure.

A study by Elmer (1977) reached different conclusions from the rest. She compared 17 abused children with 17 children matched in most aspects except for the fact that they had been referred to hospital because they had experienced accidents rather than abuse. These children were followed up at one year and eight years after the incident (in the second follow-up they were also compared with 24 children who had been neither abused nor hospitalized as a result of accidents but were otherwise matched). Elmer found no differences between the children in any of the groups with regard to emotional development. She also found no significant difference between the eight abused children who had been removed from home following the abuse incident and the nine who had remained at home. This study has raised some controversy in that the implication of the findings is that the effects of abuse of children by their parents are no worse than the effects of living in stressful and impoverished circumstances without being so abused. Elmer's (1977) study has been criticized because of its small sample size and ironically because the control group used was too closely matched to the 'abused' group:

> if an attempt was made to match for all the factors, apart from confirmed, inflicted injuries, as Elmer did in her study (1977), one might simply obtain a control group of children who were abused but not actually identified as such.
>
> (Lynch and Roberts 1982: 5)

Generally, however, studies have found that physical ill-treatment, neglect and impoverished parenting all have negative consequences on psychological development over the short- and medium-term period. As we shall see in the next section, which considers social and intellectual functioning, these consequences lay the foundation for other forms of negative behaviours on the part of mistreated and deprived children, which in turn can create further negative responses from those with whom they interact, and so on. The implications for practice are, among other things, the need to pay close attention to the emotional needs of the child as well as to his or her physical safety. Oates *et al.* (1985) argued the point convincingly:

> Although considerable emphasis is placed on supporting abusive parents to prevent further episodes from occurring, it is essential that the future emotional development of the abused child should be emphasized. As the majority of abused children remain in their natural families, they also require treatment while support is being given to their parents. This should first include a careful assessment of the child's developmental and emotional status followed by a long-term program for the child which aims at improving the child's skills in interpersonal relationships and in building up self-esteem.
>
> (Oates *et al.* 1985: 162–3)

Medium-term effects on social and intellectual functioning

The consequences considered in this section need to be seen as following on from the emotional problems outlined above. The medium-term consequences of abuse seem to have cumulative effects unless they are responded to early on.

Relationships with peers

Mueller and Silverman (1989) argue that the way in which children manage peer relationships and the experiences that they derive from them have important implications for relating to others in later life and for future mental health: 'Contemporaries increasingly seek one another as the primary sources of support, security and intimacy' (Mueller and Silverman 1989: 538). Children who have been mistreated seem to fare badly in peer relationships according to research findings (see George and Main 1979; Jacobson and Straker 1982; Hoffman-Plotkin and Twentyman 1984; Howes and Espinosa 1985; Camras and Rappaport 1993). All these studies find that physically abused and neglected children are both more aggressive and more withdrawn than their peers in play and general interaction with them. Lewis and Schaeffer (1981) concurred with these findings, but hypothesized from their study that the reason for poor social functioning on the part of abused children may not be the result of the psychologically incapacitating effects of being poorly cared for or ill-treated. An alternative explanation could be that their parents are themselves socially isolated and do not provide, or value, peer contacts for their children. There could be factors other than these that mark out ill-treated children for poor peer relationships. They could be disruptive in school (see p. 164), poorly dressed by the standards of the rest of the neighbourhood and avoided by their peers for these reasons. The effects of these experiences could be for them to react in an aggressive way or to withdraw. Most of the research in these areas has been carried out by developmental psychologists, and their focus points them more in the direction of explanations based on the effects of parent–child relationships than towards social factors. Bearing this in mind, however, there can be little doubt that abused and deprived children do not generally enjoy good peer relationships and this, therefore, can add to the difficulties they may already be experiencing in their intrafamilial relationships.

School performance

Most studies of the early school performance of mistreated children point to underachievement. Lynch and Roberts (1982) found that most of their sample performed below their IQ potential at school, the most notable deficiency being in use of language. Other studies confirm this finding (Egeland *et al.* 1983; Oates *et al.* 1984; Kendall-Tackett and Eckenrode 1996). Martin (1972) hypothesized that language delay is characteristic of abused children because of lack of trust in their environment, which in turn results in being afraid of risk-taking and acquiring little practice in speech and expressive language (see also Allen and Oliver 1982). However, as in the case of peer relationships, broader social factors may come into play. Ill-treated children may be less attractive to teachers and more demanding in terms of time. If they are aggressive or avoidant in class, they may be seen as troublesome or pass unnoticed. Knowledge of family backgrounds may lead to low expectations in terms of intellectual performance. This issue has been highlighted by research into poor educational achievements of children in care in Britain, many of whom are likely to have experienced some form of abuse (see Jackson 1996).

Two important messages come across from research into the short-term and medium-term effects of physical abuse and neglect so far reviewed. The first is that early depriving experiences can set up a cycle of events that can reinforce the ill-effects of those early events (see Howe 1995). The second, linked to the first, is that incidents of abuse, while traumatic and occasionally causing lasting physical damage and death (see p. 166), are not *per se* the major determinants of negative consequences. The ongoing climate within the family seems to be of prime importance in determining whether or not such consequences persist.

Resilient children

However, it seems that not all children are affected in the same way by similar experiences. Some children are more resilient to traumatic events and cope better than others. It was noted above that ill-treated children tend to underperform at school for a variety of reasons. However, there is some suggestion that abused children of high intelligence do reasonably well. It is argued that generally such children avoid the worst effects of abuse because they are able to understand and meet parental expectations more easily than children of lower intelligence (Frodi and Smetana 1984). Mrazek and Mrazek (1987) list 12 factors that can account for resilient survival behaviours. Most of these are associated with the child's personality and intelligence, but some are linked to situational circumstances, such as the formation of positive relationships with people outside the family and access to good educational and health facilities (see also Rutter 1985; Zimrin 1986). Lynch (1988) pointed out that although most of the children in her earlier study (Lynch and Roberts 1982) fared badly as a result of their ill-treatment, 23 per cent showed no obvious adverse effects. She drew up a profile of these survivors:

> We saw a trend for the children who were problem-free to have been identified as abused when they were young but to have escaped long-term neurological deficit. They were unlikely to have experienced perinatal problems or to have accumulated both developmental and behavioural normalities before intervention. Following intervention, although they may have been the subject of legal proceedings, these were unlikely to have been protracted or recurrent and placement changes were few. One possible protective factor identified among the abused children was the possession of above-average intelligence.
>
> (Lynch 1988: 210)

In essence, Lynch said that abuse identified early and responded to in a definite fashion is likely to result in the best outcomes, particularly if the children concerned are intelligent. Augoustinos (1987) argued that these factors are important provided the abuse is not too severe and prolonged:

> It is possible that the more severe and frequent the neglect and abuse, the less significant other factors become in affecting developmental outcome. In less severe cases, however, these factors may be better predictors of outcome than the maltreatment itself.
>
> (Augoustinos 1987: 25)

Clearly there is an implication that the responses of professionals can influence the consequences of abuse in some circumstances for better or for worse. These issues will be considered more fully in Chapter 10.

Severe psychological difficulties and impairments as a result of physical abuse

Studies have linked physical abuse with hyperactivity in children (see Whitmore *et al.* 1993) and bulimia nervosa (Rorty *et al.* 1995; Welch and Fairburn 1996). Several studies have pointed to learning difficulties as an outcome of abuse either as a direct consequence of physical injury or as a result of gross understimulation. Some care needs to be exercised in making this judgement, because (as stressed in Chapter 7), it is very difficult to disentangle whether physical abuse or learning difficulties comes first (Jaudes and Diamond 1985). Kempe *et al.* (1962) found that 28 per cent of physically abused children suffered permanent brain damage. Lynch and Roberts (1982) found that 19 per cent of their sample were mentally retarded. Lynch (1988) reviewed six US studies that showed an average rate of mental retardation among their samples of abused children of 38 per cent compared with national rates of between 10 and 15 per cent. These figures all seem to be very high. They are derived largely from hospital samples, which suggests that they are at the extreme end of the spectrum. Samples drawn from child protection registers would most probably produce much lower rates.

Another consequence of severe physical and emotional deprivation of children is the failure to grow properly. As we saw in Chapter 5, the outcome can be either short term; in the case of the 'failure to thrive' syndrome, or long term in extreme cases such as psychosocial short stature syndrome.

Longer-term pathological effects of child abuse

As was stressed in the introduction to this chapter, the longer the gap between the abusive incident and the behaviour associated with it, the greater the uncertainty about the linkage. This has already been demonstrated in the case of child sexual abuse and prostitution, and should be borne in mind throughout this section, in which the following long-term effects, which have been linked with physical abuse and neglect, will be considered: mental illness, drug-taking, delinquency and violent crime, and general life experiences and outlook.

Mental illness

Until the 1990s surprisingly little attention was paid to the connection between child abuse and later mental illness. This issue was considered briefly in Chapter 5 in the context of whether there is a link between the mental health of abusing parents and their behaviour. Here the issue is whether being abused or neglected as a child can lead to mental illness.

Carmen *et al.* (1984) analysed the case-records of 188 inpatients in a US psychiatric hospital to see if there was evidence of abuse (as children and wives) in their backgrounds. Carmen *et al.* (1984) found that 80 (43 per cent) of these patients had histories of some form of abuse; 64 of these (80 per cent) had been physically abused and half sexually abused; 72 (90 per cent) had been victimized by family members; 52 (65 per cent) were female. They argue that these figures are probably an underestimation of the real incidence of abuse in this population because they included only those cases for whom there was unequivocal evidence that abuse had occurred.

Comparisons between abused and non-abused patients showed that the former presented with more and greater problems. They generally remained in hospital for longer periods, were more likely to be alcohol abusers and were more likely to inflict injuries on themselves. They lacked self-esteem and the ability to trust, and found it hard to cope with their own aggressive impulses. Abused male patients were more outwardly aggressive, whereas abused female patients were more passive and directed their anger inwards. Carmen *et al.* (1984) stressed that there was a need to spend more time focusing on the abuse these patients had suffered as children than directly on the psychiatric illness itself.

Since this study, there have been several others supporting these types of findings. Read (1998) reported on an examination of the records of 100 consecutive admissions to an acute psychiatric inpatient unit in New Zealand. He found a lower rate of abuse than Carmen *et al.* (1984) – 22 per cent. However, patients who had been physically or sexually abused or both were more likely to be suicidal, to have longer stays in hospital and to show the most severe disturbances in symptoms and behaviour. Read (1998: 366) concluded that these findings raised 'the possibility that child abuse may have a causative role in the most severe psychiatric conditions, including those currently thought to be primarily biological in origin'.

However, there are many other possible factors apart from childhood abuse that could account for the psychiatric illnesses found in these studies, and by no means all physically and sexually abused children develop psychiatric illnesses. There are also issues relating to the definition and diagnosis of psychiatric illness. Nevertheless, many people who are treated as psychiatric patients are likely to have been ill-treated in childhood, and sensitization to this issue, along the lines suggested by Carmen *et al.* (1984) and Read (1998), can only be of benefit to them and their treatment.

Drug-taking

Cohen and Densen-Gerber (1982) studied social histories of 178 US and Australian patients being treated for drug or alcohol addiction and found that 84 per cent of them had been physically abused and neglected as children. More recently, Ferguson and Lynskey (1996) found a high correlation between young adults experiencing physical punishment as children and drug-taking, and Harrison *et al.* (1996) found a correlation between physical and sexual abuse and drug-taking adolescents. Again one must be careful in causally linking these two phenomena. Several studies of drug abuse have emphasized the cultural supports for such behaviour, rather than seeing it as a product of personal pathology (see Parker *et al.* 1988).

Delinquency and violent crime

Lewis *et al.* (1989) summarized research in the USA into the links between delinquency and child abuse. Most prospective studies showed that about 20 per cent of abused children go on to commit crimes as juveniles. Retrospective studies showed a variation of rates, ranging between 9 and 84 per cent. Lewis *et al.* (1989) reported on a longitudinal study of 411 boys conducted in Britain by West and Farrington (1977), which showed a link between harsh parental discipline and violent crime. However, as with other research into the long-term consequences of physical abuse and neglect, making causal connections is highly problematic.

Lewis and her colleagues have also carried out extensive research into violent juvenile and adult offenders and find that many have been violently assaulted themselves, frequently suffering from neurological impairments as a result, and that many have witnessed extreme violence to others in the family home. Furthermore, they argue that there is a high rate of psychiatric disturbance in the parents of violent offenders:

> Many subsequently violent individuals are raised in conditions of extreme irrationality as well as violence . . . Abuse alone does not usually create violent youngsters. It would seem that abuse, family violence and neuropsychiatric vulnerabilities in the child engender violence.
>
> (Lewis *et al.* 1989: 717–18)

These studies may be dealing with individuals at the extreme end of the spectrum and there are competing views about the generation of violence and aggression. Nevertheless, what is known about serious abuse cases in Britain suggests that some, particularly male, abusers experienced similar types of upbringing to those depicted here.[1]

General life experiences and outlook

There are very few prospective longitudinal studies of what happens to a cohort of abused children in adulthood. Nearly all the studies considered so far have been retrospective. As we saw in Chapter 7 (see

Hunter and Kilstrom 1979), such studies tend to exaggerate the connections between the behaviours being focused on and abuse.

There are two US studies that followed up abused children many years later, both of which have methodological problems. McCord (1983) carried out a record-based follow-up of children known to welfare agencies between 1939 and 1945. He traced 85 per cent of an original sample of 131 abused and 101 non-abused boys and found significantly higher degrees of alcoholism, divorce and occupational stress among the former. Those who did best from this group were those who achieved better educational performances. This study, therefore, points to the effects of abuse negatively affecting adult life. However, the study suffers from the lack of qualitative data to fill out the details of the bare facts, making it hard to know what weight to attribute to the findings.

This deficit is made up by the second study, which provides a good deal of qualitative interview-based information, but suffers from the weakness of not having a control group. Martin and Elmer (1992) followed up after 20 years a sample of 19 children who had been physically abused in the early 1960s (Elmer 1977). They found them all to be unemployed or in poor jobs, but stress that this probably reflected the economic state of the USA at this time. Their employment situation was, however, the only factor common to the whole sample. The rest of the findings present the picture of a very mixed bag. Some had poor coping skills and had undertaken very few responsibilities in their adult life; others were happily married with families. There was little evidence of aggressive interpersonal relationships, but more of general resentment towards and suspicion of outsiders and authority. Overall, there was no consistent pattern of linkage between current behaviour and early abuse.

These findings have been backed by the results of a British study by Gibbons *et al.* (1995b), who followed up 144 children ten years after they had been placed on child abuse registers for physical abuse reasons. They used a control group of a similar number of children from similar backgrounds and came to the conclusion that there was little sign that the severity of abuse had any direct effects on the child's development nine or ten years later. It is notable that Gibbons *et al.*'s (1995b) study has been used in Britain by the Department of Health (1995) to provide a note of caution about automatically responding to all physical abuse incidents as unquestionably harmful.

Summary

The studies reviewed here suffer from the problems of causally linking abuse and outcome, from weak and vague definitions of abuse and from a lack of attention to social factors as influences on behaviour, such as the differential impact of abuse on women and black people.[2]

Having noted these problems, the following general picture of the consequences of physical abuse and neglect emerges from the research that exists. Many physically abused children suffer considerable emotional and psychological problems in their early childhood, leading them to have problems in trusting other people and to suffer from a sense of personal worthlessness. Socially and intellectually they do not perform well because of this. Many physically abused children tend to be both aggressive and withdrawn; neglected children as a whole seem to be less aggressive, but are more likely to exhibit withdrawn behaviour. A relatively small number of children suffer permanently from the physical effects of injury and severe neglect. Some children seem to survive well and cope despite all the odds. Much depends on the quality of their relationships with members of their family and others during childhood and also on the individual personality and intelligence of the child in question. In the longer term, there is evidence of linkages between being physically abused and mental illness, drug abuse, delinquency and violent criminality and general adjustment to life. The connection between child abuse and these behaviours in adult lives is harder to prove, but nevertheless, particularly in the field of mental illness, the consistency of the findings are highly persuasive and have important implications for psychiatric practices.

The consequences of child sexual abuse

Research into the impact of sexual abuse on victims has been, and still continues to be, more in evidence than that into physical abuse and neglect. This stems to a large extent from the way in which sexual abuse was rediscovered in the 1980s; that is, as a result of women recounting their childhood experiences and the effects these continued to have in their adult lives. Such accounts have led to greater sensitivity to the consequences of such abuse, particularly with regard to its long-term effects. Generally, although there are the same methodological problems as in studies of the consequences of physical abuse, particularly in relation to definitional issues and the use of control groups, research into the effects of child sexual abuse seems to be more systematic and detailed. Nevertheless, there are still major difficulties in sifting out the direct impact of the abuse from that which may be attributed to other variables, such as pre-existing problems, responses to the abuse by significant adults (including professionals) and later depriving experiences.

The main overviews to be found in the literature are those by Browne and Finkelhor (1986) and Beitchman *et al.* (1991, 1992). The studies reviewed by these writers differentiate between short-term and long-term

effects and this is the structure used here. After a review of the main
findings of research into these two types of effects, consideration will
be given to key variables that are thought to have an important influence on the extent and severity of the consequences.

Short-term effects of child sexual abuse

The research on the short-term effects of sexual abuse is not as well
developed as that in relation to the long-term effects. Beitchman *et al.*
(1991) pointed out that only 1 of the 49 studies reviewed by Browne
and Finkelhor (1986) is an empirical study of children with a control
group. Studies making up this deficiency since 1986 have been in
greater supply, but the net result of the findings is disappointing for
those who would like to build intervention and short-term treatment
approaches on the basis of research information.

Browne and Finkelhor (1986) preferred the term 'initial effects' to
'short-term effects' because the latter suggests that such effects do not
persist, which may or may not be the case. They defined 'initial effects'
as those which become evident in the first two years after the known
onset of the abuse. Beitchman *et al.* (1992) made the important point
that there may be long-term effects without short-term effects first
having been apparent.

The following behavioural and emotional responses have been found
to be evident in the short term.

General psychopathology

Gomes-Schwartz *et al.* (1990) studied 156 sexually abused children
treated by a family crisis programme in New England, USA. They
assessed these children on a variety of emotional and behavioural
criteria, and compared them with children referred to them for reasons
other than sexual abuse and also with similar aged children in the
general population. On overall ratings, severe psychopathology was
higher for children of all ages who had been sexually abused than it
was for children living in the community. For the 7- to 13-year-old
group, who were generally more vulnerable than abused preschool
children and older adolescents, the degree of difference was as great
as 40 per cent. However, in comparison with other patients at the
centre, the degree of overall psychopathology was slightly less.

Fearfulness

Browne and Finkelhor (1986: 149) stressed that 'the most common
initial effect noted in empirical studies is fear'. Gomes-Schwartz *et al.*
(1990) found that 45 per cent of their most vulnerable group of children

(the 7- to 13-year-olds) were experiencing fearful reactions to what had happened to them within the first six months following the onset of abuse. Browne and Finkelhor (1986) found rates as high as 83 per cent in a study by De Francis (1969). However, Beitchman *et al.* (1991) pointed out that similar degrees of fear and depression (see next section) are to be found in general psychiatric populations and, therefore, the emotions attributed in these studies specifically to sexual abuse could be linked to other stress-inducing factors.

Depression, withdrawal and suicide

Friedrich *et al.* (1986) found from a sample of 61 sexually abused females that 46 per cent were experiencing a range of internalized emotions including depression within two years of being abused. They also found that a withdrawn reaction was more common in younger victims. Anderson *et al.* (1981) found that 25 per cent of females who had been sexually abused showed symptoms of depression afterwards. Calam *et al.* (1998) in a study of 144 child sexual abuse cases reported in Liverpool found that 36 per cent were experiencing anxiety and depression nine months after intervention and that this number had reduced only slightly after two years. Koreola *et al.* (1993) found high levels of depression in a sample of 39 sexually abused 6- to 12-year-olds, but concluded that the depression was not linked to the severity of abuse. The sample included many children with mild learning difficulties who had been exposed to a range of stressful events in their brief lives. Other studies have also pointed to depression in school-age sexual abuse victims resulting from tendencies to internalize problems (Kolko *et al.* 1988; Goldston *et al.* 1989). Lindberg and Distad (1985) found that one-third of their clinical sample of 27 adolescents with incest histories had attempted suicide.

Hostility and aggression

Some victims of child sexual abuse respond by directing anger and aggression outwards. This response is more common among adolescents. Gomes-Schwartz *et al.* (1990) identified angry reactions in between 45 and 50 per cent of the 7- to 13-year-olds in their sample, and Calam *et al.* (1998) reported anger as a response in one-third of their sample after nine months. Friedrich *et al.* (1986) found that children aged from 6 to 12 were more likely to externalize their feelings than younger children. Gomes-Schwartz *et al.* (1990) pointed out that there are problems associating aggressive reactions purely with sexual abuse because many of the children in their sample were also subjected to physical violence or the threat of it. Thus the aggression they displayed could have been a result of this rather than of the sexual abuse they experienced.

Low self-esteem, guilt and shame

The findings with regard to low self-esteem as a short-term consequence of sexual abuse are rather mixed. De Francis (1969) reported that 58 per cent of victims expressed feelings of inferiority. However, Gomes-Schwartz et al. (1990: 88) found that their preschool age sample of sexually abused children 'exhibited a more positive self-concept than the normative population'. This finding held true for the older age groups as well. Conte and Schuerman (1987) reported on the adverse effect that guilt can have as victims mature, but there is no evidence of such guilt among preschool children (Lusk and Waterman 1986), which is as we would expect, given the social nature of this emotion.

Physical symptoms

Browne and Finkelhor (1986) reported on clinical studies that find an association between sexual abuse and subsequent sleeping and eating disorders. Calam et al. (1998) found that one-third of their sample experienced sleep problems and about one-fifth were soiling and wetting nine months after the initial investigation. However, Gomes-Schwartz et al. (1990) reported that relatively few school-age children in their sample exhibited serious somatic complaints. Beitchman et al. (1991) argued that such behaviours are as common in general psychiatric populations and, therefore, could be associated with factors other than sexual abuse.

Running away and other 'acting-out' behaviours

Running away from home has been associated with sexual abuse of adolescents in several research studies (Meiselman 1978; Herman 1981). Silbert and Pines (1981) found that 96 per cent of female prostitutes who had been sexually abused as children were runaways. Other 'acting-out' behaviours associated with sexual abuse are truanting, drug and alcohol abuse and promiscuity. Not all studies, however, support such connections (Johnston 1979; Goldston et al. 1989).

Cognitive disability, developmental delay and school performance

Gomes-Schwartz et al. (1990) found relatively high rates of both cognitive disability and developmental delay in their preschool sample. They are careful not to see these problems as consequences of sexual abuse, speculating that they may have existed before abuse took place and may have contributed to these children's vulnerability to such abuse. The school performance of the abused 7- to 13-year-olds was significantly worse than for the general population, a finding supported by Tong et al. (1987), but again there are problems in linking this specifically to sexual abuse. It is notable that Calam *et al.* (1998) found that one-third of the children in their sample were experiencing school difficulties nine months after intervention and one-quarter were experiencing problems with peer relationships.

Inappropriate sexual behaviour

Precocious and excessive sexual behaviour in sexually abused children is widely reported on by both parents and professionals and confirmed by studies of children playing with anatomically correct dolls (Jampole and Weber 1987; Sivan *et al.* 1988). Gomes-Schwartz *et al.* (1990) reported that 27 per cent of 4- to 6-year-olds who had been abused exhibited excessive sexual behaviour and 36 per cent of 7- to 13-year-olds. Deblinger *et al.* (1989) found high rates of sexually inappropriate behaviour in a sample of 155 children, as did Friedrich *et al.* (1986). Beitchman *et al.* (1991) felt that the variation in rates should lead to caution in making assumptions that sexual abuse is necessarily a precursor to inappropriate sexual behaviour in children. Nevertheless, this linkage is clearer and stronger than that between sexual abuse and any of the other factors so far considered. However, there is still a major problem with regard to children as they get older, that is that of deciding what constitutes appropriate or excessive sexual behaviour.

Summary

Two conclusions can be drawn from this brief review. The first is that while an appreciable number of sexually abused children do experience behavioural and emotional problems in the two years following abuse compared with children who have not been abused, the linkage between these behaviours and sexual abuse is weak and other factors could account for them. As Beitchman *et al.* (1991) stressed:

> We do not know whether many of the symptoms reported in the literature are specific to sexual abuse or whether they are attributable to other factors such as the child's pre-morbid level of functioning or a disturbed home environment. The contribution of these preexisting constitutional and familial factors to observed psychopathology needs to be more carefully examined.
>
> (Beitchman *et al.* 1991: 552)

The only relatively clear direct outcome is that of inappropriately sexualized behaviour, which occurs in between 25 and 33 per cent of all sexually abused children.

The second conclusion is that sexual abuse *per se* does not have an incapacitating effect in the short term for most children. Browne and Finkelhor (1986: 164) pointed out that 'In the immediate aftermath of sexual abuse one-fifth to two-fifths of abused children seen by clinicians manifest some noticeable disturbance.' It should be stressed that this apparently strange conclusion may result from the fact that a broad definition of sexual abuse is used in most of the studies including, for instance, various degrees of seriousness and both intrafamilial and extrafamilial abuse. It should be noted that the timing of the research is also important: Calam *et al.* (1998) found that their sample of children was experiencing far more problems two years after the abuse incident than they were at four weeks afterwards.

However, which children do suffer most will become clearer when consideration is given later in this chapter to variables such as violent abuse and abuse by a close and trusted relative. It has to be stressed that research into this area is still new and experimental; it is important, therefore, to interpret the findings carefully and not to draw hasty conclusions from them at this stage.

Long-term effects of child sexual abuse

Many of the behaviours and emotions discussed in relation to short-term effects of sexual abuse are also to be found in studies of long-term effects. As stressed at the start of this chapter, the linkages, seen to be problematic in the case of short-term effects, are even more problematic with regard to long-term effects because of the greater length of time between the abuse and the observed behaviour and because of the possible effect of a much wider range of intervening variables.

Fear and anxiety

Briere (1984) is reported in Browne and Finkelhor (1986) to have found that women sexually abused as children were twice as likely as non-abused women to experience fear, anxiety and nightmares and three times as likely to experience difficulties sleeping. However, a complicating factor in terms of a specific linkage with sexual abuse is that 49 per cent of his sample had also experienced physical violence as children and women. Beitchman *et al.* (1992: 106) came to the following conclusion on this linkage: 'While anxiety symptoms among adult women appear to be associated with CSA, it is not clear that this effect is independent of force or the threat of it.'

Depression and suicide

Beitchman *et al.* (1992) reviewed eight studies and found that six reported an association between child sexual abuse and depression as measured by either self-rating or psychiatric diagnosis. Fromuth (1986) did not find a connection, but the average age of her sample was 19.4

years whereas most of the other studies involved older women. With regard to suicide, studies are more equivocal in their findings. Disentangling cause and effect is again a problem; suicide attempts and thoughts seem to be most closely linked to women who have experienced physical violence as well as sexual abuse as children.

Self-esteem

Browne and Finkelhor (1986: 156) pointed out: 'Although a negative self-concept was not confirmed as an initial effect, evidence for it as a long-term effect was much stronger'. Bagley and Ramsay (1986) report a low self-esteem rate of 19 per cent among women sexually abused as children and 5 per cent among their control group. Herman (1981) reported that 24 (60 per cent) of her clinical sample of 40 female victims of incest had negative self-images compared to 10 per cent of her control group.

Likelihood of revictimization

Russell (1986) found that 65 per cent of women sexually abused as children were victims of subsequent or attempted rape, compared with 36 per cent of non-abused women. She also found that between 38 and 48 per cent had been subjected to physical violence by husbands and partners compared with 18 per cent of the control group. Briere (1984), as already stated, found that 49 per cent of his sample of women abused as children had been violently assaulted by men as adults. Various reasons have been put forward for the association of child sexual abuse and subsequent abuse, ranging from increased vulnerability in the case of girls leaving home as a result of their abuse experiences, to psychological needs to have their feelings of low self-esteem reinforced by further ill-treatment.

Sexual disturbance

As we have seen, sexualized behaviour was the short-term effect most closely related to child sexual abuse. Consideration has already been given to the questionable link between prostitution and child sexual abuse. Research shows there is a connection between being abused as a child and problems with sexual behaviour in adult life. There are difficulties in evaluating the validity of this research in that sexual problems are not clearly defined and there may well be high levels of sexual dysfunction or dissatisfaction in the general non-abused population. However, clinical studies such as those of Meiselman (1978) produce very high rates of sexual difficulties (87 per cent), and non-clinical studies, with the exception of Fromuth (1986), find significantly higher rates among their abused samples than among non-abused controls. Adams *et al.* (1995) found very high rates of sexually inappropriate behaviour among mentally ill children and adolescents with histories of being sexually abused.

Psychiatric problems and sexual abuse

There is some evidence to link child sexual abuse with personality disorder in adults (see Beitchman *et al.* 1992: 109), but as yet the link is weak. The link between child sexual abuse and mental illness has already been referred to in the section on physical abuse (Carmen *et al.* 1984). Other studies, specifically looking at sexual abuse, have confirmed these earlier findings. Wurr and Partridge (1996) in a study of 120 patients admitted to a psychiatric hospital in England found a 46 per cent rate of sexual abuse, whereas only 14 per cent had been revealed under the normal assessment procedures. Gold *et al.* (1996) found in a sample of 135 women in an outpatient treatment programme that severity and duration of abuse, along with low age at onset of abuse were factors that were associated with more deep-seated psychological problems at a later age. Briggs and Joyce (1997) in New Zealand have reported high rates of post-traumatic stress disorder among a sample of 73 women attending a counselling programme. There was a particularly close association with multiple abusive episodes which involved sexual intercourse.

Other long-term consequences of sexual abuse

Linkages have been found between eating disorders and sexual abuse (Waller 1994; Welch and Fairburn 1996), drug and alcohol misuse (Peters 1976; Herman 1981; Briere 1984; Harrison *et al.* 1996) and, as noted in the introduction to this chapter, prostitution. Finally, it should not be forgotten that there are physical consequences of sexual abuse. Jaudes and Morris (1990) collected data from a sample of 138 sexually abused children referred to hospital between 1979 and 1987 and found that one-third of them had a sexually transmitted disease. Their average age was just over 6 years old. Although, despite their name, it is possible for sexually transmitted diseases to be passed on in non-sexual ways, the chances of this are very small (Neursten *et al.* 1984). Some deaths are also closely linked to sexual abuse. Most of these are extrafamilial, but there are cases of deaths being associated with extrafamilial abuse as well (O'Hagan 1989: 72–3).

Summary

During the 'rediscovery' of child sexual abuse in the 1980s, considerable emphasis was placed on its long-term incapacitating effects, based on individual studies and case accounts. The findings of research into the general long-term effects confirm that women who have been sexually abused are more likely than women who have not to have problems in later life with regard to fear, anxiety, self-esteem, depression, satisfactory sexual relations and general mental health, and to be vulnerable to further abuse. However, such consequences are not inevitable.

Browne and Finkelhor (1986) estimated that less than one-fifth of sexually abused women evidence serious psychopathology, but stress that this fact should not be used to minimize the seriousness of child sexual abuse. In the section that follows, the focus will be on factors that can be influential in creating the worst outcomes.

Variables affecting both short- and long-term consequences

Seven variables have been associated in the literature with influence on the harmful effects of child sexual abuse: age at onset of abuse; sex of child; degree of seriousness of the abuse; duration of abuse; relationship of the abuser to the abused; abuse accompanied by violence; and the way in which the abused child was helped and responded to at and after the time of disclosure.

Age at onset of abuse

Throughout the preceding sections, the age of the child at the onset of abuse has been referred to because clearly some reactions are age-specific or development-specific. It is generally believed that both the short- and long-term consequences of sexual abuse are less harmful the younger the children, because of their lack of awareness of the social stigma attached to sexual abuse. Gomes-Schwartz *et al.* (1990) (see p. 171) found that their 7 to 13 years age group experienced more adverse reaction than did children in their 4 to 6 years and 14 to 18 years groups. Adams-Tucker (1981) found that children first abused after the age of 10 experienced worse short-term symptoms than did those first abused before this age. By contrast, Russell (1986) found that longer-term ill-effects were more likely to be experienced by those first abused in pre-puberty rather than in adolescence. Beitchman *et al.* (1991) suggested that age needs to be considered in conjunction with other variables. It could be that many children discovered to have been abused in early childhood may not have suffered the adverse effects of a long period of abuse or have been subjected to as much violence, as they are unlikely to resist as strongly as older children, and that these factors could account for the less traumatic effect rather than age *per se*.

Sex of child

Overall, there is not enough research in this area to come to definite conclusions. Abuse of girls and boys can take different forms and this may account for different outcomes rather than the fact that the victims are boys or girls. Pierce and Pierce (1985) reported that boys are more likely to be subjected to violence when being sexually abused and, therefore, more likely to suffer negative effects. On the other hand, girls are more likely to be abused by their natural fathers and to be removed from home following abuse, both factors being associated to some extent with negative outcomes. It is possible that sexually abused boys are more socially stigmatized than sexually abused girls because of the relative rarity of such abuse and its threat to masculine assumptions. This too could increase negative effects.

Degree of seriousness of the abuse

The research findings linking severity of abuse (measured by type of abuse, such as whether it was penetrative or not) with harmful consequences are not consistent. Browne and Finkelhor (1986) referred to ten studies that considered both long- and short-term effects of abuse of different degrees of severity. Six of these found that there was a link between harmful outcomes and the severity of the abuse; four found no significant link. They concluded: 'Thus it is premature to conclude that molestation involving more intimate contact is necessarily more traumatic than less intimate contact' (Browne and Finkelhor 1986: 169). Beitchman *et al.* (1992) argued that the studies quoted by Browne and Finkelhor (1986) as not proving an association did not include enough serious abuse on which to make a proper judgement. They looked at some additional studies and concluded that there is a linkage between serious abuse and trauma as perceived by the victim, but a less strong association between such abuse and objectively measured mental health.

Duration of abuse

Browne and Finkelhor (1986) reviewed eleven studies that measured the link between duration of abuse and trauma. They found that six confirmed that the longer the abuse went on, the more traumatic was the effect on the victim, whereas five did not. They did not differentiate between short- and long-term effects. One might expect there to be similar short-term responses to abuse of long and brief duration, and Gomes-Schwartz *et al.* (1990) confirmed this. Beitchman *et al.* (1992) argued that abuse of longer duration is associated with longer-lasting harm. They stressed that the picture can be distorted by the impact of violence. There are many instances of one-off abuse accompanied by violence, which can have traumatic effects on victims. If this is allowed for, then the link between duration of abuse and long-term harmful effects is stronger than Browne and Finkelhor (1986) suggested.

Relationship of the abuser to the abused

Clinical accounts suggest that the more closely related the abused child is to the abuser, the greater is the degree of harm likely to result. Thus intrafamilial abuse is likely to have a more harmful effect than extrafamilial abuse, and abuse perpetrated by a natural father more than that perpetrated by an uncle. Browne and Finkelhor (1986) found that several studies that compared all intrafamilial abuse with all extrafamilial abuse concluded that the harmful effects were the same. They attribute this unexpected finding to the fact that extrafamilial abuse is more likely to be accompanied by fear and that some relatives who abuse may be less trusted than, say, a neighbour with whom the abused child might normally have more interaction. However, abuse by father figures compared with that by all other perpetrators was considered to result in greater trauma. Beitchman *et al.* (1992) concurred with this finding, pointing to gross betrayal of trust as the reason for the degree of trauma or lasting harm created. They also pointed out that such abuse is likely to be of longer duration and to reflect and create considerable family dysfunction.

Abuse accompanied by violence

Browne and Finkelhor (1986) considered the use of violence or the threat of it as the most important factor contributing to both short- and long-term distress and harm. The study by Russell (1986) provided a good example of the closeness of the association between these two variables. All those who reported violent abuse experienced extreme or considerable trauma, as did 74 per cent of those who experienced forceful abuse. Of those who experienced non-forceful abuse, 47 per cent experienced lasting harm.

Response to abuse

Gomes-Schwartz *et al.* (1990) found that a negative (for example non-believing) response by a parent or parents to a child's allegation of sexual abuse was associated with greater short-term psychopathology on the part of the child. It exacerbated the already existing problems. Conte and Schuerman (1987) found that a supportive response from the family was an important factor in reducing the extent of long-term problems following sexual abuse. Beitchman *et al.* (1991, 1992) referred to several other studies that confirmed the influence of family response on both short- and long-term harm. Their view was that victims of child sexual abuse are more likely than non-victims to come from disturbed families and, therefore, that they are particularly likely to be responded to by their families in a negative way. Clearly this argument is more relevant to intrafamilial abuse. Also of importance in this area is the response of professionals to allegations of sexual abuse. Elwell and Ephloss (1987) found that bad handling of intervention by the police and other professionals was associated with increased short-term trauma. Gomes-Schwartz et al. (1990) found that children removed from their families showed the most short-term problems but, as Browne and Finkelhor (1986) comment, these might have been the most problematic cases in the first place.

There seems, therefore, to be reasonable evidence to suggest that sexual abuse is likely to be most harmful in the following instances:

- where the abusive act involves penetration
- where the abuse has persisted for some time
- where the abuser is a father-figure
- where the abuse is accompanied by violence, force and/or the threat of it
- where the response of the family is negative.

While the age and sex of the abused child have some impact on the outcome, the research does not provide clear indications of the direction of these variables' effects. There is not sufficient information on the impact of professional intervention to evaluate conclusively its effect for good or ill.

Concluding comments

For some health and welfare practitioners, the degree of detail of all this research may seem unnecessary, in that child sexual abuse of the type in which they frequently become involved – largely intrafamilial and often of a very serious nature – clearly has harmful effects on the child. It can seem to be somewhat hair-splitting to separate which element of abuse in a generally abusive situation causes the most harm. Similarly, research which suggests that children who are removed from families do less well than those who remain can be frustrating when it is apparent that removal is the only feasible course of action. Nevertheless, there are some important and relevant findings, namely that sexual abuse of children is not necessarily incapacitating for them in later life. There is a tendency among professionals to make this assumption, which can in itself have negative effects.[3] In particular, awareness of the impact of the variables just discussed is an important starting-point for assessing the consequences for the child and how to organize a response. Such knowledge provides a framework for intervention, not a blueprint. Children whom one would expect to suffer less harmful effects on the basis of known research findings may in fact experience considerable trauma. As has been repeatedly stressed, there are weaknesses in the research, and findings need to be carefully interpreted. Nevertheless, despite its limitations, this is the best formal available knowledge and it should, therefore, have relevance for policy and practice in this field.

Recommended reading

Beitchman, J., Zucker, K., Hood, J., Da Costa, G. and Akman, D. (1991) A review of the short-term effects of child sexual abuse, *Child Abuse and Neglect*, 15: 537–56.

Beitchman, J., Zucker, K., Hood, J. *et al.* (1992) A review of the long-term effects of child sexual abuse, *Child Abuse and Neglect*, 16: 101–18.

Browne, A. and Finkelhor, D. (1986) Initial and long-term effects: a review of the research, in D. Finkelhor *et al.* (eds) *A Sourcebook on Child Sexual Abuse.* Beverly Hills, CA: Sage.

Erickson, M., Egeland, B. and Pianta, R. (1989) Effects of maltreatment on the development of young children, in D. Cicchetti and V. Carlson (eds) *Child Maltreatment: Theory and Research on the Causes and Consequences of Child Abuse and Neglect.* Cambridge: Cambridge University Press.

Gibbons, J. Gallagher, B., Bell, C. and Gordon, D. (1995) *Development after Physical Abuse in Early Childhood: A Follow-Up Study of Children on Child Protection Registers.* London: HMSO.

Gomes-Schwartz, B., Horowitz, J. and Cardarelli, A. (1990) *Child Sexual Abuse: The Initial Effects.* Beverly Hills, CA: Sage.

chapter **ten**

RESEARCH INTO CHILD
PROTECTION PRACTICE

The aim of this chapter is to analyse what research tells us about the way in which health and welfare professionals respond to child abuse and the effectiveness of this response.

Prior to the early 1990s, the amount of research into British child protection practice was very limited. There were very few studies of the work of mainstream statutory agencies (see Dingwall *et al.* 1983; Corby 1987; Waterhouse and Carnie 1992). Child protection public inquiry reports gave glimpses of practice approaches, but as such inquiries were held when things appeared to have gone wrong, they formed a rather skewed sample. There were more, but still relatively few, accounts and evaluations of intervention into physical and sexual abuse cases by voluntary agencies and in hospital settings (Baher *et al.* 1976; Lynch and Roberts 1982; Dale *et al.* 1986; Ben-Tovim *et al.* 1988) and a few accounts of action research projects (Smith and Rachman 1984; Browne and Saqi 1988). Overall, there were very few studies of the effectiveness of child protection interventions, only a small amount of research into the consumer end with regard to parents (Brown 1986; Corby 1987) and no formal research data about the views of children.

The picture has changed considerably since the mid-1990s. As pointed out in Chapter 4, following the report of the Cleveland inquiry (Butler-Sloss 1988), the Department of Health commissioned a wide range of studies into various aspects of the child protection system; these reported in 1995 and 1996. The following key areas of child protection practice were among those studied: responding to referrals (Gibbons *et al.* 1995a), carrying out investigations (Cleaver and Freeman 1995; Farmer and Owen 1995), involving parents in the initial stages of intervention and at child protection conferences (Thoburn *et al.* 1995), inter-professional collaboration (Birchall with Hallett 1995) and responding to sexual abuse allegations (Sharland *et al.* 1996). Each of these studies had an evaluative element in them; importantly, most of them gathered information from parents and children, to some extent filling the consumer perspective gap referred to previously. Since these studies, there have been several others into parental and child involvement in the child protection process (see Corby and Millar 1997; Marsh and Crowe 1998) and child sexual abuse investigations (Corby 1998).

It should be stressed, however, that while we now have a clearer picture of how the British child protection system operates as a result of this research, we still lack information about preventive measures, treatment initiatives and about what works and what does not.

In general terms, the USA has produced more in the way of evaluative studies than in Britain. It established the National Center on Child Abuse and Neglect in the 1970s to promote research initiatives in this field. Even so, there is much concern about the lack of knowledge development about effective intervention (see Melton and Flood 1994; Oates and Bross 1995).

Studies and accounts of practice will be considered in the following way. First, those relating to prevention and prediction will be examined. Second, the focus will be on studies and accounts relating to assessment and decision-making at the early intervention stage and later in the process, when important long-term plans are being considered. Third, consideration will be given to treatment issues and, finally, general effectiveness studies will be examined.

Prevention and prediction

Prevention

Prevention of child abuse has not been a popular topic of research. While many commentators agree that prevention is the most constructive approach to the problem of child abuse, examples of ways of achieving this are very limited. Gough (1993) considered this issue and found that there are three types of preventive strategies: those targeted at the whole population, such as community education programmes; those targeted at certain communities, usually those afflicted by poverty and deprivation; and those targeted at certain groups of families in which children are considered to be at risk.

With regard to the first type of preventive strategy, Gough (1988) found little evidence of abuse awareness campaigns in Britain. The main exceptions to this are educational programmes in schools aimed at equipping children to protect themselves against sexual abuse. Gillham (1991: 48–63) provided a useful overview of such programmes and research related to them. He questioned their effectiveness, which has generally not been rigorously tested. Most programmes of this kind tend to focus on extrafamilial abuse, and one study demonstrated that they have only limited impact (Kelly et al. 1991). In the USA, Finkelhor et al. (1995) found from a study of 2000 children that victimization prevention instruction, as they termed it, can increase knowledge among children and the likelihood of disclosure.

The second strategy involves lay and professional people operating in community centres to provide general help and support with parenting for any family in a particular geographical area. Such projects are often headed by voluntary societies, and the focus is on general child care problems rather than specifically on child abuse (see Holman 1988). This type of preventive (or supportive) work is not widespread in Britain. It should not be confused with family centre work, which tends to be more focused on child abuse issues and is not, strictly speaking, preventive, because it usually follows on from abuse incidents being reported. Following the shift to a more family supportive approach to child protection in the mid-1990s, this type of prevention may become more common. It is more characteristic of other European countries such as Belgium, the Netherlands and Germany. Thyen *et al.* (1995) provided a good example of this in their report on the Child Protection Center in Lübeck, Germany, which works on a supportive and voluntaristic basis with families where child maltreatment is a concern.

The third strategy involves selecting out certain types of parents who are considered to be potentially abusive to their children for extra support from nursing or medical staff. This type of selective or predictive approach has received a good deal of attention, particularly by the medical profession. Some reference has already been made to predictive studies in Chapter 5, but they will now be considered in greater detail.

Predicting child abuse

The idea of predicting abuse is an attractive one because of its preventive potential. It also has financial appeal because it raises the possibility of targeting limited resources on those areas where they are most needed and most likely to be effective. However, there are considerable problems associated with the predictive approach in practice, as the following studies and critiques of them show. In the USA, Kempe and Kempe (1978) reported on a study in which 350 mothers and their new-born babies were screened for child-abuse potential. On the basis of interviews and observations around the period of giving birth, 100 mothers were rated as 'high-risk' and 50 as 'low-risk'. Fifty of the 'high-risk' mothers were followed up after two years and it was found that eight of their children had been placed on child protection registers compared with none of the low-risk group. Five of these eight children had been hospitalized with serious injuries. In addition, the high-risk children were significantly more likely to have undergone accidents in the two years and their parents were more likely to be considered 'abnormal'. On the basis of these findings, the authors claimed to have successfully predicted 79 per cent of all incidents of abuse that took place during this period, that is 75 out of 95.

Both Parton (1985) and Montgomery (1982) subjected this study to close scrutiny and were critical on three main accounts. The first is that the definitions used for abusive behaviour are very loose and wide-ranging. As we have seen, they included accidents in the home and 'abnormal parenting'. Montgomery (1982) pointed out that only the eight cases that were registered should properly have been considered abusive, a view which, if accepted, drastically reduces the high rate of accurate prediction claimed by Kempe and Kempe (1978). The second issue is that even if one uncritically accepts the 79 per cent

Table 10.1 Factors associated with child abuse in Browne and Saqi (1988)

1 Parent indifferent, intolerant or overanxious towards child.
2 History of family violence.
3 Socio-economic problems such as unemployment.
4 Infant premature, low birth weight.
5 Parents abused or neglected as a child.
6 Step-parent or cohabitee present.
7 Single or separated parent.
8 Mother less than 21 years old at time of birth.
9 History of mental illness, drug or alcohol addiction.
10 Infant separated from mother for greater than 24 hours post-delivery.
11 Infant mentally or physically handicapped.
12 Less than 18 months between birth of children.

positive prediction rate, this still means that 21 per cent of parents were wrongly suspected of abusing their children, the implications of which will be considered below. Third, 20 of the 95 cases of abuse were missed.

Parton (1985) reported on a study in Bradford by Lealman *et al.* (1983), who used maternity records to predict the likelihood of abuse (measured by the much narrower criterion of child protection registration). In all, 28 children out of a total of 2802 were registered, of whom 17 were predicted. However, although the researchers predicted nearly two-thirds of the eventual abusers, in so doing they wrongly predicted 483 others, a false positive rate of 28 to 1! With regard to intervention, Lealman *et al.* (1983) found that specialist social work input did not significantly affect family functioning or, in contrast to the findings of Gray *et al.* (1977), influence the rate of serious abuse.

Browne and Saqi (1988) reported on a series of predictive studies carried out with health professionals in the Surrey area. Using a 12-item checklist (see Table 10.1) at birth and after one month on a population of 14,238 families, they identified 949 of these as high-risk. However, the results after two years were disappointing in terms of successful prediction – only 1 in 17 (6 per cent) had abused their children (no definition of abuse given).

Dingwall (1989) subjected prediction studies similar to this carried out at the Park Hospital in Oxford to close scrutiny (see Lynch and Roberts 1977, 1978; Ounsted *et al.* 1982). Dingwall (1989) found that these studies all had weaknesses because they employed vague definitions of child abuse and because the criteria on which the predictions were based are questionable. Dingwall's view is that parents from lower social classes are more likely to be predicted as potential abusers because they are more likely to be identified as troublesome at an early stage by health professionals. In addition, he pointed out that the fact that the definitions of abuse used by the researchers are very general and include concerns linked to parental non-cooperativeness means that all that is being predicted is that families originally perceived as troublesome continue to be seen as such:

> There may be a simple circularity here: the record of noncompliance predicts future non-compliance which is likely to precipitate the labelling of a child as abused, but which has no established relationship to the actual treatment of the child.
>
> (Dingwall 1989: 40)

In summary, these studies demonstrate that it is possible to predict between 65 and 80 per cent of known future abuse. On the debit side, however, is the fact that in this process at least 20 per cent of any sample are likely to be wrongly thought to be likely to abuse or neglect their children, and if one uses an official narrower definition of child abuse the rate of false prediction soars to a much higher level. Therefore, these studies fail in their aims of accurately targeting those families who might benefit from specialist help. In addition, they provide little in the way of information about the best way to prevent the abuse they predict.

It is not only the effectiveness of the predictive approach that is in question. There are also major questions about the ethics of this sort of activity. Is it, for instance, ethical to make an assessment of potential parental care without informing parents of what is happening? Is it ethical not to inform parents about concerns resulting from this assessment? It is not clear from these studies whether parents had any awareness of the fact that they were being assessed in this way. The only justification for this lack of openness can be that secrecy is essential in order to ensure the well-being of the child. There is, however, no evidence that lack of candour is likely to improve the safety of the child. Working with parents on the basis of shared concerns may be a more effective strategy in achieving this goal.

In concluding this section on prediction, it should be stressed that there is little evidence of maternity screening and service targeting of this kind taking place in mainstream practice in Britain. Only in exceptional cases where parents have previous histories of child abuse or where there are obvious signs of problems on maternity wards (including serious drug misuse) are families subjected to special scrutiny at the time of the birth of a child. Otherwise screening is left to the wit, experience and training of community health professionals. This system can be both effective and non-stigmatic because of its universalist base. However, to work well, such services need to be well resourced and workers need to be well trained in the issues surrounding child abuse and well integrated with other, particularly welfare, services. In the USA, there was an upsurge of interest in home visiting programmes in the 1990s (see Leventhal 1996). Some of the programmes

Table 10.2   Finkelhor's Risk Factor Checklist (1979)

1 Stepfather present
2 Separated from mother
3 Not emotionally close to mother
4 Mother did not complete high school
5 Low family income
6 Lack of physical affection from father
7 Mother sexually punitive
8 Having two or fewer friends

described there, while not being clear about the ethical issues just referred to, do seem, if properly resourced, to have the potential to both help families and reduce risk.

A final point to be made about predictive work is that it has been used mainly in the area of physical abuse and neglect. Predicting the likelihood of sexual abuse in this way has so far not figured so highly on the agenda. The exception is Finkelhor's Risk Factor Checklist (1979) (see Table 10.2) which has proved of limited effectiveness (see Bergner *et al.* 1994).

Assessment and decision-making

The practice of assessment in child protection work clearly has some links with the preceding section on prediction, in that its function is to make plans for the future on the basis of what is known about a family's past and present in the light of available research knowledge. There are two key assessment points in child protection work: when abuse first comes to light and there is a need for short-term decision-making; and when there is a need to decide on the action required to ensure the longer-term future protection and well-being of the child. The former will be considered in this section and the latter in the next.

Short-term decision-making at child protection case conferences

The lack of detailed research into short-term assessment and decision-making in child protection cases makes it hard to know how it is actually carried out. Officially such assessments are drawn up at inter-disciplinary case conference settings. However, there are important decisions reached before this stage, particularly those about whether allegations or suspicions of abuse are of sufficient seriousness to warrant case conferences. Gibbons *et al.'s* (1995a) research shows that only one-quarter of all child protection referrals result in conferences being held. However, this study does not tell us which cases are filtered out of the system and why. We are forced, therefore, to rely on what takes place at the conference stage of intervention to develop our knowledge about assessment in the early stages of intervention.

Research studies carried out by Hallett and Stevenson (1980), Dingwall *et al.* (1983), Dale *et al.* (1986) and Corby (1987) all commented critically on standards of assessment at case conferences in the late 1970s and early 1980s. Hallett and Stevenson (1980) made much of inter-professional defensiveness and dysfunctional group processes as impediments to good early assessment and decision-making. Dingwall *et al.* (1983) came to the conclusion that most assessments made at case conferences were, for a variety of structural reasons, including inter-professional conflict, likely to result in an under-estimation of the degree of risk to a child. Dale *et al.* (1986) considered that there were grave dangers of professionals becoming polarized over case conference decisions and exacerbating already existing difficulties. Corby (1987), while finding little inter-professional disagreement over cases of serious abuse, reported a good deal of confusion in more marginal cases about why some children were registered and others were not. Decisions did not seem to be reached on the basis of a rational assessment of the degrees of risk (see also Campbell 1991).

Studies in the 1990s have confirmed this rather negative picture. Higginson's (1992) research suggested that decision-making is still not based on a close assessment of potential risk. To a large extent she attributed this to the weakness of the research knowledge base that is available to provide guidance in this area. Farmer and Owen (1995) showed how conferences serve the needs of professionals to demonstrate their accountability. There is still much controversy about whether risk should be assessed by the use of checklists based on research, and this will be discussed further in the next section on long-term assessment. In short-term assessments, such information does not seem to be explicitly used by professionals, though research suggests that, implicitly, factors such as the seriousness of the abuse, the cooperativeness of the parents and histories of previous abuse all play some part in the process (Medden 1985; Corby and Mills 1986). Murphy-Beaman (1994) pointed to the dangers of using risk assessment schedules as part of initial assessments:

> Accurate predictions of violence are considerably more difficult to make for individuals who have not yet clearly behaviorally demonstrated harmful acts, but only show an apparent proneness for such acts. This would be the case with many parents who are suspected of being at risk for child abuse.
>
> (Murphy-Beaman 1994: 194)

Sexual abuse

The research and practice so far discussed have been concerned mainly with physical abuse and neglect. Short-term assessment in the field of child sexual abuse has followed a very different line. The focus of such assessments has been much more on children than on adults. This has come about because there are few observable signs of child sexual abuse and, therefore, the main means of assessing whether or not a child has been sexually abused or is likely to be is via the child's testimony. While indicators of sexual abuse have been devised (see Finkelhor 1979; Porter 1984), they tend to be used as supportive evidence to a child's testimony. Similarly, physical evidence of sexual abuse, following events at Cleveland, tends to be used as supportive rather than main evidence. However, securing a child's evidence has proved to be a highly controversial matter (see Chapters 3 and 4). In Britain, following the events in Cleveland and the Orkneys, a system was devised to produce evidence which was suitable for criminal proceedings in a way that was not intrusive for the child concerned. This involves joint interviews with police and social workers (see Fielding and Conroy 1992) and medical examinations in appropriate cases. The net result of these changes has been to limit the amount of assessment that can take place at the early stages of child sexual abuse investigations. More in-depth early assessments focused on children have been actively discouraged. Thus, for example, the use of methods involving anatomically correct dolls has diminished considerably despite reports of positive applications in research carried out in the USA (Everson and Boat 1994). Two points are worth noting. First, children do not often reveal the full truth about being sexually abused to order. Shapiro Gonzalez *et al.* (1993: 288) pointed out: 'Clinicians treating child abuse victims must understand that disclosure is a continuous process and be aware that some aspects of the abuse may not be revealed until months into therapy.' Second, the shift towards more evidence-focused intervention under the Memorandum of Good Practice has not been very effective. According to a Social Services Inspectorate (1994) report, only 6 per cent of all interviews were used in criminal proceedings.

The context of initial child protection assessments

Early assessments in child protection work often take place in stressful and hostile circumstances (see Farmer and Owen 1995) and, therefore, opportunities for calm and careful analyses of situations are relatively rare (see Corby 1996). In situations of extreme hostility, such assessments can be carried out only with the backing of the courts. This was the thinking behind the introduction of Child Assessment Orders under section 43 of the 1989 Children Act, which empowers social workers to carry out assessments in situations where parents are denying them access to a child, though they have in fact been rarely used (see Dickens 1993). Another approach to facilitating early assessments in conflict situations has been to remove suspected abusers from the household. Under schedule 2.5 of the 1989 Children Act, local authorities are empowered to defray the expenses of an alleged abuser living away from home pending the outcome of an investigation. Under the 1996 Family Law Reform Act, courts may, on making an interim care order, enforce the removal of a parent from the family home provided the remaining parent is in agreement.

Summary

Research into and accounts of short-term assessment and decision-making in child protection work point to a different approach being adopted depending on whether the subject of inquiry is a case of physical or sexual abuse. In the former, assessment tends to focus on the parents and in the latter on the children. In the case of physical abuse and neglect, there is little evidence of use of research findings in carrying out assessments, and some evidence to suggest that this is justified. Initial assessment practices in child sexual abuse have been considerably altered following the events of the late 1980s and early 1990s. There has been a shift towards the gathering of practical evidence and away from more child-centred approaches.

Despite these differences, there has been some cross-fertilization between the assessment approaches in physical and sexual abuse cases. More attention is now paid to the child's testimony in physical abuse and neglect cases, and greater consideration to assessing the broader family needs in sexual abuse cases.

Longer-term assessment and intervention

The bulk of cases that come into the child protection system involve moderate abuse and low standards of child care (see Thorpe 1994). In most of these cases decisions are reached to monitor families, provide support services and review progress at a later date. As we saw in Chapter 4, recognition of the fact that concerns about this type of abuse or neglect dominate child protection work has led to much greater encouragement of a more family supportive approach. The Department of Health (2000b) has published new assessment guidelines which reflect this shift. These contain three areas of emphasis: the needs of the child, the capabilities of the parents and the material and social environment in which the family is situated. The focus is much less on identifying abuse and risk of it, and much more on meeting the needs of the child and the family. This is in sharp contrast to the assessment guidelines, known as the Orange Book, published over a decade earlier

(DoH 1988), which reflected the then prevalent concern with risk of serious abuse.

The current Department of Health (2000b) guidelines are arguably less informative than their predecessor on how to assess families where there are concerns about serious abuse or risk. These cases are the focus in this section, where there is need to take important decisions about the long-term future of children who have been previously subjected to serious abuse, or who are thought to be at risk because of previous serious abuse of siblings or because their parents have been convicted or suspected of previous serious abuse. While these cases may form only a small percentage of all those referred, nevertheless, the consequences of inadequate assessment can be disastrous. Difficult decisions have to be reached about whether it is best for children in these situations to remain with or, since in such cases emergency removal is likely to have occurred, return to their parents and, if so, under what circumstances, with what services and safeguards.

Physical abuse

In the field of physical abuse and neglect, this has perhaps been the most pressing issue of all. In most of the cases publicly inquired into, the main concerns have not been the effectiveness of initial assessments and interventions; the Darryn Clarke inquiry (DHSS 1979) and the Kimberley Carlile inquiry (Greenwich 1987) are the most notable exceptions.[1] Most of the children in public inquiry cases have died while legally in the care of or under the supervision of the authorities, but actually living at home with their parents. The focus of concern has been whether these children should have been allowed to stay with their parents or have been returned to their parents' care, and whether the supervision they received was of a reasonable standard.

Generally the practice of the statutory agencies has been heavily criticized for being too parent-centred in its thinking in this area and for not being sufficiently thorough in its assessments. It is with cases such as these that risk assessment schedules (discussed on p. 190) are thought by many to be most effective. Such schedules were first brought to professionals' attention in the late 1980s.

Greenland (1987), whose work is also referred to in Chapter 5, devised a checklist (see Table 10.3), derived from analysis of 100 child deaths by abuse in Canada, which he recommended for use in making long-term decisions about children who had been seriously abused.

Earlier in the 1980s, a whole plethora of risk assessment schedules had been developed in the USA. There have been many concerns about such schedules. The main ones, identified by Wald and Wolverton (1990) are, first, that while variables like those identified by Green-land (1987) may be associated with serious child abuse, the nature of

Table 10.3   Greenland's high-risk checklist (1987: 185)

For parents
1 Previously abused/neglected as a child.
2 Age 20 years or less at the birth of first child.
3 Single-parent/separated; partner not biological parent.
4 History of abuse/neglect or deprivation.
5 Socially isolated; frequent moves; poor housing.
6 Poverty; unemployed/unskilled worker; inadequate education.
7 Abuses alcohol and/or drugs.
8 History of criminally assaultive behaviour and/or suicide attempts.
9 Pregnant, postpartum or chronic illness.

For children
1 Was previously abused or neglected.
2 Under 5 years of age at the time of abuse or neglect.
3 Premature or low birth weight.
4 Now underweight.
5 Birth defect; chronic illness; developmental lag.
6 Prolonged separation from mother.
7 Cries frequently; difficult to comfort.
8 Difficulties in feeding and elimination.
9 Adopted, foster-child or stepchild.

the association is not clear. Greenland (1987: 171) stresses that 'it seems reasonable to assume a high-risk situation exists when an infant has suffered a serious non-accidental injury and more than half the check-list items, in any order, are checked'. Yet, there is no proof that simply adding up variables to reach a score in this way is likely to result in an accurate assessment of risk. There may well be some combinations of variables indicative of greater risk than others; at present, we simply do not know. Second, these factual indicators need to be considered alongside knowledge about the dynamic interaction within the family; taken on their own, they are insufficient. Third, checklists are no substitute for clinical or professional experience. They are best used as an aid to making decisions.

Checklists and risk schedules have not been much used in Britain despite the great outcry about child deaths for nearly two decades following the publication of the Maria Colwell inquiry report (DHSS 1974). To some degree there has been a distrust, particularly by social workers, of using knowledge derived from public inquiry reports in any systematic way (see Corby *et al.* 1998). Most recently (as noted in Chapter 4), there has been an increase in interest in some circles prompted partly by concerns about the shift towards a family support approach (see Bridge 1998).

Much of the research about rehabilitation of seriously abused children is derived from medical settings and is pessimistic about the effectiveness and advisability of this course of action. Hensey *et al.* (1983), for instance, argued that the children who best survived their experience after being taken into care were those for whom an early decision was made to sever parental contact and to place the child permanently with a substitute family. King and Taitz (1985) came to a similar conclusion with regard to children failing to thrive. Lynch and Roberts (1982) were also doubtful about the value of rehabilitation unless it is accompanied by individual therapy for children. In their study they found that re-injury was rare, but that the development of the children remained at a low level after they had returned to their parents.

Dale *et al.* (1986) carried out a study of their work at the Rochdale NSPCC Special Unit and came to more positive conclusions about the potential for successful rehabilitation. In their work, they used techniques derived from strategic family therapy to assess parents whose children had been removed from home following abuse, and to decide whether rehabilitation was a safe prospect. Their work was based firmly on having therapeutic control. They argued that most abusing parents denied or minimized the abuse done to their children and that there was a need not only to make them understand why they abused their children but also for them to accept full responsibility for their actions. Failure to achieve these goals usually resulted in a decision not to return the child to the parents. The unit found that 65 per cent of children from 26 families were initially rehabilitated to their parents; 10 per cent of these children were subsequently returned to care. There were no re-injuries (over an unspecified time period) among those children who remained at home. Monitoring and follow-up were considered necessary only at a minimal level.

Another study with implications for successful rehabilitative work was reported on by Farmer (1992). Case records of a sample of 150 abused and neglected children placed home-on-trial were studied to see what factors were associated with success or failure; 45 per cent of placements were considered to be beneficial to the children and 19 per cent detrimental. Abuse or neglect reoccurred in just over 25 per cent of all cases. Successful rehabilitation was seen to be linked to purposeful social work involvement, planning and regular visiting. It was also linked to the number of placements that the child had experienced while in care. Those who had been placed with only one foster-parent did better than those with more than one placement. It could be that these were the least problematical cases in the first place. However, what this study demonstrates is that social workers in mainstream services can achieve successful rehabilitations without attempting to bring about major changes in parental attitude. They need to select the cases with the best prospects, have regular direct contact with families and work purposefully and in a planned way to achieve rehabilitative goals.

Sexual abuse assessments in statutory agencies

With regard to longer-term assessments in serious sexual abuse cases, Corby (1998) found little formal activity or systematized assessment taking place. Often there was little opportunity for carrying out formal assessments because abuse continued to be denied sometimes throughout long periods of involvement. As with short-term assessments, the difficulties of trying to analyse situations characterized by conflict and deception should not be underestimated. Similar findings were reached by Sharland *et al.* (1996). Waterhouse and Carnie (1992) found that the main factors taken into account in deciding on a child's protection needs in cases of sexual abuse were the response of the non-abuser to the abused child, the age of the children and their degree of assertiveness and ability to protect themselves in future. All these studies were into the work of local authority social workers.

Another finding that all these studies reached was that little or no work is done by statutory-based workers in relation to adult abusers. The main concern with regard to them is the threat that they might pose to children and the main solution adopted is to find means of ensuring that they are separated from the children concerned.

The Great Ormond Street approach

The picture is somewhat different in hospital and voluntary agency-based services. Ben-Tovim *et al.* (1988) devised a form of assessment, based on family therapy principles, that involved all members of the family. They argue that intrafamilial abuse is a product of faulty family functioning and is sustained by secrecy, and therefore that it is a prerequisite to successful treatment that family members communicate openly with each other about what has happened in the past and what they wish for the future. This entails abusers admitting to all their family members what they have done and the opening up of emotional blockages. Openness and explicitness are seen as essential counters to the secrecy that has helped to maintain the abusive situation, and they must be achieved regardless of the pain and anxiety created in the process (Furniss 1991). Often by the stage at which this assessment is carried out the family has broken up, usually as a result of a prison sentence being imposed on the abuser. This form of assessment requires family attendance at monthly meetings over a period of 12–15 months and is supplemented by children and parents attending separate groups or in some cases receiving individual therapy. Ben-Tovim *et al.* (1988) conducted a follow-up (no time period specified) of families who were assessed between 1981 and 1984 (55 per cent of the families completed the full course of assessment). They found that 83 of 120 children (69 per cent) had not been reabused, whereas 19

(16 per cent) had, and it was not clear whether reabuse had taken place in the remaining cases. Most of the family make-ups had changed by the time of follow-up. After their prison sentence 15 per cent of abusing parents had returned home.

Clearly Ben-Tovim *et al.*'s (1988) work has similarities with that of Dale *et al.* (1986) in the case of physical abuse. Both studies focused on the need for full acknowledgement of the abuse. Both see faulty family dynamics as at the root of abuse and both merge assessment to a large extent with therapy. Both also require considerable time, resources and expertise. Both control the inflow of work, in terms of type and quantity of cases worked with. Clearly statutory agencies cannot under current circumstances replicate this sort of assessment practice, particularly given the growth in child sexual abuse discovery since the late 1980s (see Chapter 6). The issue for policy-makers is, if approaches of this kind are seen as desirable, who should implement them and how they should be resourced.

Summary

In overview, the picture of longer-term assessment and decision-making in the child protection field is as follows. With regard to physical abuse and neglect, statutory agencies do not follow a particular theory, and generally, unlike the situation in the USA, the use of risk assessment schedules is not popular. State social workers in Britain operate under a philosophy that oscillates between a preference for rehabilitation where possible in the belief that ultimately a child is better off in its own family and a preference for non-rehabilitaton as the safest course of action in terms of the protection of the child. Assessments and decisions are frequently based on the actions of parents after the abuse and, particularly, on their cooperativeness and desire to retain the care of their child. Some research shows a reasonable degree of success with rehabilitation (Dale *et al.* 1986; Farmer 1992). Other research, particularly that carried out by the medically oriented professions, points to clean-break approaches being more beneficial for children.

With regard to sexual abuse, the lack of formal theory-based assessment, in statutory social work is also evident. Before Cleveland, there is evidence that such social workers were applying approaches, methods and knowledge derived particularly from the USA. To a large degree this type of work has been seen as too intrusive and too narrowly focused on the child, and is now relatively rare. In longer term assessments, social workers seem to be less likely to favour rehabilitation with the continuing presence of an abuser in the household than is the case in physical abuse and neglect. Ben-Tovim *et al.'s* (1988) approach in a specialist setting has been more optimistic in relation to rehabiliation and demonstrated some success.

Providing treatment and support

Generally research suggests that there is a lack of treatment provided for children who have been abused and their families. Clearly, there are exceptions; the assessment work of Ben-Tovim *et al.* (1988) obviously involves a good deal of therapeutic input as well. However, particularly in the case of children who have been physically abused and neglected, direct forms of treatment or therapy have been found to be lacking, often because the focus is on working with parents to ensure that they are more responsive to their children's needs (see Greenwalt *et al.*, 1998). Despite the fact that there is greater sensitivity about the needs of children who have been sexually abused, research evidence points to a lack of provision of therapeutic services. Humphreys (1995) in an Australian study found that 56 per cent of children received counselling despite a policy of providing such a facility for all sexually abused children. Tingus *et al.* (1996) reported slightly larger numbers receiving counselling in California. They found that white children were more likely to be counselled than black children, as also were children who were removed from their families. The picture in Britain with regard to therapeutic inputs is even more dismal. Sharland *et al.* (1996), Corby (1998) and Calam *et al.* (1998) all reported very low levels of child-focused treatment. Corby (1998) in a study of 40 child sexual abuse cases dealt with by statutory agencies in the north-west of England commented as follows:

> As far as the children were concerned, only a few offers of therapeutic help either in the form of group or individual work were made, and by no means all of these were taken up. Selection for, and allocation of, therapeutic help was a very hit-and-miss affair, depending on the availability of resources, knowledge of them by social workers and openness to them by both children and parents.
>
> (Corby 1998: 135)

It should not be concluded from this that there are no therapeutic facilities for sexually abused children across Britain (see Lindon and Nourse 1994). The concern is that excellent projects of the kind they describe are rare.

Therapeutic work with adults in child abuse cases is somewhat more in evidence in physical abuse cases than in sexual abuse cases, but even here the emphasis is more on support and monitoring (see Farmer and Owen 1995). Family centres have played an increasingly central role in this aspect as well. There is less evidence of therapeutic work with adults in cases of child sexual abuse. Hooper (1992) has highlighted the needs of mothers of children who are abused in this way, and Sharland *et al.* (1996) and Corby (1998) found that there were sensitive and supportive responses to mothers by social workers, particularly if they were themselves deemed supportive of their own children. Adult abusers are largely excluded from child protection interventions in Britain. If convicted of sexual offences against children, there are programmes run by probation officers or in the prison setting which are aimed at breaking down denial and getting offenders to accept responsibility for their actions. In the USA (Giaretto 1981), the Netherlands (Frenken 1994) and Belgium (Marneffe 1996), there are opportunities to provide therapeutic intervention services for certain abusers instead of criminal prosecutions. Frenken (1994) stresses that in the Netherlands, such interventions are possible only for first-time offenders, who did not use violence in their sexual acts and who would otherwise have been given short prison sentences. This seems to be a sensible attempt to differentiate between types of abusers, but adoption of this sort of approach is unlikely in Britain in the near future because of the current social concerns about paedophiles.

There has been much more attention paid to the treatment needs of young sexual abusers (see Erooga and Masson 1999) in Britain. Two considerations have driven this: the first is that such offenders are children and many may have been subjected to abuse themselves, and the second is that intervention at this stage may prevent them from becoming recidivist paedophiles and placing other children at risk.

The effectiveness of intervention and treatment

Some reference has already been made to the effectiveness of professional intervention into child abuse in the previous sections; in particular the work of Ben-Tovim et al. (1988), Dale et al. (1986) and Farmer (1992) provided some positive intervention outcomes. In this section we consider a broader range of British and US studies. Before doing so, there are some important issues to consider in measuring effectiveness. The first relates to the indicators of success or failure. Several researchers (Lynch and Roberts 1982; Calam and Franchi 1987) have argued that non-recurrence of abuse is not an adequate measure because, as they have found, the emotional quality of care for a child may continue to be low even though he or she is no longer subjected to physical violence. Second, there is the issue of the length of time allowed between intervention and the measurement of outcome. Most studies follow up cases within two years at the most, which may be too short a time to measure lasting effects. Third, there is the problem of establishing causal links between intervention and outcome in that both successful and unsuccessful results could be the consequence of variables that have nothing at all to do with the intervention programme.

Physical abuse and neglect

Therapy for parents

Evaluations of therapeutic approaches in physical abuse and neglect are rare in Britain; the work of Dale *et al.* (1986) has been noted. There have also been some small-scale behavioural approaches which have reported some success (see Bourn 1993; Iwaniec 1997) and, as we saw in Chapter 8, some that have reported failure (Smith and Rachman 1984).

Generally, however, there is a stronger tradition of evaluation in the USA. Kempe and Kempe (1978), reporting on therapy with parents who had physically abused their children, found a 20 per cent outright failure rate, that 40 per cent were considered to have grown and developed into more mature and positive individuals and carers, and 40 per cent, while not achieving this form of change, at least did not reabuse their children.

Green *et al.* (1981) reached similar findings. In a study of 79 parents who had seriously abused their children, they found that intensive psychotherapeutic help led to some improvement in 40.5 per cent of the sample, by which they meant that they had learned to control their aggression and not reabuse. Significant improvement, including the development of greater insight into themselves and the development of empathy and understanding of others, took place in 27.8 per cent of the sample. The remaining 32 per cent showed no change in their behaviour and attitudes: 16 per cent had reabused their children at follow-up and it was not clear whether reabuse had happened or not in the remaining 16 per cent. They found higher rates of success among parents who stayed longer in treatment. Other factors related to treatment failure were the seriousness of the effects of the abuse and parents having gross misperceptions of their children's level of maturity and undertanding.

Cohn and Daro (1987) reported on the evaluation of federally funded projects set up between 1970 and 1980 to develop treatment-based responses to the problem of physical abuse and neglect. Most of these projects were based on the approach pioneered by Kempe and Kempe (1978). However, they did not achieve the same rates of success. While in treatment, rates of reabuse reported ranged between 30 and 47 per cent. Overall, 42 per cent of parents treated were thought to have reduced potential for neglect, but high drop-out rates were common. Cohn and Daro (1987) were of the view that overall the results are disappointing and pointed to the need to focus more on prevention than treatment.

Jones (1987) in a review of British and US studies focused on those families that do not respond to treatment and that he terms 'untreatable'. These include those who have carried out serious forms of abuse, such as non-accidental poisoning, burns, neglect resulting in psychosocial short stature syndrome and cases attributed to Munchausen's syndrome by proxy. Other factors associated with untreatability are parents who were severely maltreated themselves as children, parents with personality disorders or suffering from psychotic illness, parents who deny abuse, lack empathy and drop out of treatment programmes. The problem with this type of list is that it is too baldly stated and, therefore, as it stands, of little use in the world of practice, where there is an expectation that parents will be at least considered for a second chance. While there may have been a tendency for social workers to have been overcommitted to rehabilitation in the past, there are also dangers in unequivocally labelling people as untreatable. For instance, is it justifiable to view parents who drop out of programmes as being untreatable as a result? Clearly there is a need to examine the nature of the programmes to see if they have played a part in the outcome, independent of the parents' personality.

Other approaches

On a more positive note, Cohn and Daro (1987) found that the more successful programmes were those that did not rely exclusively on individual therapy but had a range of other inputs, including community support schemes of the kind reported on by Gough (1988) in Britain, groupwork inputs including the work of Parents Anonymous and parent education classes.[2] Cohn and Daro (1987) also found that programmes which used temporary substitute care or ensured the removal of the perpetrator were among the most successful.

Some studies have demonstrated good levels of effectiveness in day nursery/family centre provision. Culp et al. (1987) in the USA report significant improvements in a range of social, physical and psychological skills among a group of 35 3-year-old children attending a therapeutic day centre compared with a control group receiving normal services. The input was intensive and a range of services was provided, including individual and group therapy for parents and children, which was supplemented by a crisis line and other community supports. The importance of involving parents is highlighted in a US study by Crittenden (1983), which suggested that more traditional approaches, which use nurseries as forms of stress-relieving respite care, do not seem to be effective.

A study by Gabinet (1983a) also raised some important questions about day centre work. She examined the issue of treatment drop-out in relation to a child protection focused family centre in Cleveland, Ohio, which provided support for mothers, group activities and some parental education. She found that of 100 families referred to the centre in 1979, 53 failed to attend despite being given three appointments. Another five families were seen fewer than five times. Gabinet (1983b) argued that the failure of the family centre she studied was due to the fact that its focus on child protection was seen as threatening and unhelpful by those assigned to it. She advocated a more general child-care oriented service with more power being shared with parents using such centres. Ong (1985) pointed to similar concerns in a study of an NSPCC family centre in Britain.

A related issue is the notion of compulsory treatment. Does it work? The findings of US studies on this subject are somewhat mixed. Rivara (1985) reported higher completion rates where court orders apply, as did Wolfe *et al.* (1981). However, Green *et al.* (1981) found that court-ordered treatment was negatively correlated with successful outcome. Gabinet's (1983a) study did not include court-ordered cases, but she found that over half of those families who had been sent to the centre with the threat of their children being removed if they refused did not attend.

These issues are relevant to the British scene in that there has been much more use of family centres in the late 1980s and 1990s. Treatment at such centres is not legally enforceable without parental consent, but it may be that many parents feel they have no option but to attend if they wish to continue caring for their children. Unfortunately, there has been little or no evaluation of these issues and their impact on effectiveness.

Summary

Studies into the effectiveness of a wide range of intervention methods in the USA suggest that individual counselling or psychotherapy for parents seems to have some influence on outcomes in terms of improved general care of children and in terms of re-injury rates. Overall, however, the results are not as good as the initial work of Kempe and his associates suggested (Kempe and Kempe 1978). Providing supplementary forms of help and support, such as community help, group and crisis line support, improves the effectiveness of individual therapy. Imposing treatment on unwilling clients seems to result in mixed outcomes. There is some support for the view that programmes that involve and empower parents are more effective. Where and in what circumstances compulsion is effective or necessary remains to be seen.

While it has been argued that there has been a dearth of evaluative studies in Britain, it should be noted that some of the DoH-sponsored studies which reported in 1995 and 1996 do contain a general evaluative element. In relation to physical abuse and neglect, Thoburn *et al.* (1995) and Farmer and Owen (1995) found that the rate of reabuse over a two-year period of abused and neglected children was 30 per cent. They studied children coming through the child protection system in circumstances where neither they nor their parents received particular therapeutic intervention; the main focus of intervention was on making arrangements to ensure that children were not exposed to further risk. A high percentage of the parents felt stigmatized by the way in which interventions were carried out.

Sexual abuse

There have been several studies evaluating the effectiveness of sexual abuse interventions in terms of the likelihood of reabuse and in terms of the perceptions of children and parents about professional intervention. As regards general effectiveness, studies of specialist centres in Britain and the USA using family therapy techniques to inform intervention and assessment (Giaretto 1981; Ben-Tovim *et al.* 1988) have reported high rates of success. The 20 per cent reabuse rate in Ben-Tovim *et al.*'s (1988) study has already been mentioned. Giaretto's (1981) study of interventions into 600 families in the 1970s reported that 90 per cent of children removed from their families being rehabilitated in less than a month after placement and no reabuse at all. He rather vaguely stated that the re-establishment of normal father–daughter relationships was achieved in most families.

Studies of general statutory social work interventions into child abuse cases have found higher levels of reabuse. Sharland *et al.* (1996) reported a 30 per cent rate of reabuse. Corby (1998) estimated that 35 per cent of children in his sample remained at risk of abuse when the cases were closed by the child protection professionals.

It seems, therefore, that the specialist agencies have higher success rates, with the US approach described by Giaretto (1981) performing best of all. These differential rates of success could be explained in many different ways. It is worth noting that Ben-Tovim *et al.* (1988) and Giaretto (1981) selected cases to work with, unlike the statutory agencies in the studies by Sharland *et al.* (1996) and Corby (1998), which were required to deal with all referrals made to them. The type of family or problem being worked with could have been very different in these studies. Giaretto (1981) reported that the clients were largely white and middle class, whereas the majority of those in the other three studies were from the lower social classes. Finally, there is the effect of cultural and institutional differences. In comparison with the climate in which Giaretto (1981) was operating, the British response to intrafamilial sexual abuse seems punitive and over-controlled by the police and criminal law.

Gomes-Schwartz *et al.* (1990) reported on the effectiveness of their crisis intervention approach with children who have been sexually abused. They found that their approach was beneficial for over three-quarters of their clients and, above all, served the important function of laying good foundations for later involvement. Roberts and Taylor (1993) in a study of 60 children who had been at the receiving end of sexual abuse investigations reported that, although they had found the process of intervention traumatic, most were glad with hindsight that it had taken place. Berliner and Conte (1995) in the USA reached a similar conclusion with a sample of 82 children:

> The children's comments on disclosure confirm that it is an extremely difficult decison to make. They describe wanting to tell, but having many fears about the reactions of others. They make it clear that their suffering does not end with telling. It is heartening that in spite of this, they are virtually unanimous that it is the best course of action. They believe that their emotional recovery and stopping the abuse, both of themselves and others, will only occur if it is reported.
>
> (Berliner and Conte 1995: 383)

Gomes-Schwartz et al. (1990) also found that many of the families they worked with had many other problems, which were seen to need a wider range of long-term supports and help, a finding echoed by Sharland et al. (1996) and Corby (1998). Gomes-Schwarz et al. (1990) also argued that treatment programmes must recognize parents' needs for support and that collaboration between treatment and child protective services is essential for successful outcomes. Sharland et al. (1996) found that only 24 per cent of the parents in their study had positive feelings about the way in which intervention had been handled.

There were considerable developments in the management and treatment of sex offenders in Britain in the late 1980s and 1990s. Most of this took place in and around the criminal justice system, and apart from the work of Ben-Tovim et al. (1988) and a few others, took place with individual offenders outside the context of the family. The report of the Association of Chief Officers of Probation (1996) found that there were strategies in place for managing adult sex offenders in 98 per cent of probation services. There are also a growing number of non-statutory approaches (see Morrison et al. 1994). Studies of effectiveness are few in number. Furby et al. (1989) provided an overview of the effectiveness of such treatment programmes in Britain and the USA and came to the rather pessimistic conclusion that there is no evidence that they reduce the reoccurrence of sex offending. Erooga and Masson (1999) provided more optimistic evidence in relation to young sexual abusers, except in the worse cases characterized by long histories of being abused themselves in childhood, high levels of anti-social behaviour and aggression, and low social competence.

Concluding comments

Studies of the effectiveness of interventions into child sexual abuse cases produce a variety of results, and great care must be taken in using the findings because of the methodological problems associated with linking inputs and outcomes in this most complicated field of study. Bearing this in mind, it seems that with regard to achieving reasonable protection for children following sexual abuse, the specialist more family-focused approaches are the most successful. Nevertheless, statutory intervention achieves a 70 per cent success rate in terms of prevention of reabuse. Children by and large appreciate the outcomes of intervention, whereas parents tend to see it as intrusive and not as helpful as they would wish it to be. With regard to therapeutic work with adult offenders the jury is still out, but there are signs of more effective work taking place with young abusers.

Recommended reading

Browne, K. and Herbert, M. (1997) *Preventing Family Violence*. Chichester: Wiley.

Cicchetti, D. and Carlson, V. (eds) (1989) *Child Maltreatment: Theory and Research on the Causes and Consequences of Child Abuse and Neglect*. Cambridge: Cambridge University Press.

Waterhouse, L. (ed.) (1993) *Child Abuse and Child Abusers: Protection and Prevention*. London: Jessica Kingsley.

chapter eleven

CURRENT ISSUES IN CHILD PROTECTION WORK

In this chapter attention will be focused on some of the key issues currently being debated by researchers and practitioners in the field of child protection in Britain, the USA and mainland Europe.

First, the general picture. The 1990s saw considerable developments in child protection policy and practice in Britain and the USA. In both these countries, after a period of almost unparalleled growth of interest in, and broadening of the definitions of, child abuse, there has been a considerable reshaping of thinking in part as a consequence of the sheer numbers of cases resulting from these developments. Since the mid-1990s in Britain, the focus has moved away from the protection of children by direct intervention towards the provision of greater family support as a means of reducing abuse and neglect. In the USA, there has been a shift towards more targeted preventive work in the shape of greater use of early risk assessment and home visiting programmes.

The European response has been quite different. This is largely because the upsurge of interest in and focus on child abuse which took place in Britain and the USA in the 1970s and 1980s did not take place elsewhere in Europe to the same extent. Child protection systems of the kind developed in Britain and the USA (and also in Canada, Australia and New Zealand) have not been developed. Less directly child protectionist, more family supportive approaches have characterized the responses to dealing with child abuse problems in countries like France, the Netherlands and Germany since the 1960s. To some degree, there has been a questioning of this more indirect approach among European nations, and there is some admiration of the more overt approaches adopted in Britain. The differences in approach persist, but as a result of European unity there is beginning to be more dialogue between Britain and other European nations about child protection policies than there was at the end of the 1980s (see Pringle 1998).

In parts of the world so far unmentioned, intrafamilial child abuse remains low on their list of priorities: street children and children in substandard institutions dominate concerns in parts of Eastern Europe and South America. In many parts of the southern hemisphere, child prostitution and child labour are also major concerns.[1] In such countries rife with poverty and deprivation, as was true of Britain in the late nineteenth century, abuse of children by their parents is a relatively minor concern. It should be noted that these concerns are not confined to these countries; concerns about institutional abuse, runaway and homeless children and child prostitution were causes of much concern in Britain at the end of the 1990s. However, the scale of these problems is quite different compared to that which faces poorer countries.

Within this general context, the following areas seem to be most pressing for those concerned with child protection in Britain:

- balancing child protection and family support
- working at a societal level to prevent child abuse
- developing therapeutic services for abused children and adults
- responding to offenders.

Balancing child protection and family support

Achieving what is considered to be a reasonable balance between working supportively with parents to tackle child care and neglect problems and protecting children from risk of abuse and neglect became (as we have seen) the key issue in child protection work in Britain in the second half of the 1990s (Parton 1997). It is clear from a study of the history of state intervention into families to protect children, that this is not a new issue, but rather a perennial one. The state is heavily reliant on the family to socialize children, and is extremely wary of intervention for this reason. Donzelot (1980) showed how the state in France in the early twentieth century developed strategic means of supporting the family by focusing on mothers as the key carers and by a shift away from directive to psychotherapeutic methods of influence. Similar developments took place in Britain, and child care practice from 1948 to the end of the 1960s was heavily influenced by maternal deprivation theories and casework intervention with families.

A return to more direct intervention into families followed from the realization that children were subject to abuse within the family: the concept of child abuse replaced that of child neglect, and working with parents was replaced by a greater concern to protect children from them. Rising affluence and greater sensitivity to the needs (and rights) of children lay at the core of this development. As we have seen, however, social work intervention into the family ultimately came to be seen as excessively intrusive, particularly in the case of sexual abuse. The result has been a shift away from a direct intervention approach to a more indirect family supportive emphasis.

It is clear from recently published guidelines (DoH 2000a) that this shift does not represent a complete turn-round or reversion to the approaches of the 1960s. The situation is much different now; awareness of child abuse in a broad variety of forms is widespread, and society is still highly concerned about child abuse, even though its focus seems to be less on abuse within the family and more on institutional abuse and extrafamilial sexual assaults. Thus, child abuse is still high on the agenda of government guidelines, but it is required to be seen within the context of families in need of support. Child protection practitioners are expected to distinguish early on between referrals that require a family supportive approach and those where there may be a need for more authoritative intervention resulting in processing through the child protection system. In both cases, despite the different emphases, they are required to try and achieve some form of balance between the broader needs of the families and the children's needs to be protected.

In many ways, these developments are positive ones. The research summarized in the *Child Protection: Messages from Research* publication (DoH 1995) clearly demonstrated that many families referred for general child care concerns received little supportive help because the focus of child protection was firmly on identifiable abuse. However, the reason for this state of affairs seems to have been placed firmly at the door of child protection professionals; put simply, they were seen as being too narrowly focused on child abuse, too defensive in their practices and unable to recognize that children's needs and standards of care were inextricably linked to their wider family situations. There seemed to be little awareness that these responses were an almost inevitable outcome of over two decades of pressure to focus more exclusively on the protection needs of the children. There also seemed to be a lack of realization that child care resources were limited and that focusing them on the worst cases (that is those where children were thought to be most at risk of abuse) was a reasonable strategy in the circumstances.

Currently, therefore, social workers and other child protection professionals are being required to use far more discretion and judgement in their assessment of child care and child abuse referrals than before. They are required to assess the needs of families and to provide supportive packages, and where they decide to process cases through the child protection system they are required to work in partnership with parents and to involve them more fully in the decision-making process. Again these are positive developments, but there are some major problems.

First, the shift in approach is unlikely to be achieved without considerable retraining for social workers and other professionals, because it is likely to create uncertainties for individual practitioners and for inter-professional liaison. It has taken many years to achieve reasonable, but still less than perfect standards of interagency work (see Birchall and Hallett 1995). By trying to achieve a better balance of child protection and family support, some of the more established certainties may suffer and open up the possibility of a return to some of the problems of poor inter-professional communication so commonly cited in child abuse inquiries in the 1970s and 1980s (see Corby *et al.* 1998).

Second, the more balanced approach seems to have considerable implications for resources. Most of the families referred as a result of child care and child abuse concerns are families living in poverty with considerable material problems and difficulties. There has been little consideration of the cost implications of meeting the needs of these families in order to support them in their care of their children. Recent developments in social security policy, tax and child care incentives are evidence of the Labour government's determination to tackle poverty by means of job incentives and higher rates of employment. There seems to be little indication that the kinds of supportive approaches being encouraged in current child care policy are in keeping with this government's broader philosophical approach to the problems of social exclusion. In this context, the indirect approach to tackling child abuse concerns may well promise far more than it delivers.

Finally, there is the issue of child sexual abuse and family support. While it is clear that most of the child sexual abuse cases dealt with by the statutory child care sector are from deprived families with a wide range of material and other problems, there are some particular difficulties in combining family support and child protection in these cases. Sexual abuse allegations create powerful tensions within families and between parents and child protection professionals. All too often, the events are shrouded in secrecy which may be maintained by threats and there is usually strong resistance to any form of professional intervention. While alleged abusers remain in the same households as children in circumstances such as these, it is extremely difficult to operate in a family supportive way. The same argument also applies to other types of abuse where families are similarly resistant.

Overall, there is little doubt that achieving a balanced approach between child protection and family support is an important goal; indeed it has always been so (see Ferguson 1990). The concern at present is whether sufficient thought has been given to what a balanced approach entails in relation to different sorts of cases, and to the cost implications of such an approach. In addition, there seems to have been insufficient consideration given to whether the child protection system currently in operation can be well enough adapted to achieve the required balance, and whether the sort of training both for individual professionals and for professionals working together is adequate to equip them for this more complex task.

Working at a societal level to prevent child abuse

While much of the child abuse research considered in this book focuses on individuals and families where things have gone wrong and tries to locate the problem within these microsystems, it is clear that society as a whole carries much responsibility for the existence of child abuse. At the most, it creates the climate for such mistreatment to persist and, at the least, it fails to tackle the conditions in which it can thrive and to thereby prevent it.

There can be little doubt that much more could be done at the societal level to reduce the extent of child abuse. In the previous section, the impact of resources, poverty and social exclusion has already been considered. These are basic issues that lie at the heart of a great deal of child abuse and neglect as currently defined. While it is true that many economically poor parents do not neglect their children and that child abuse (particularly sexual) is not confined to the poorer social classes, the alleviation of poverty would go a long way to lay the foundations for a society free from child abuse. It should be noted that poverty does not relate simply to finances, but to educational opportunities, and health and leisure facilities as well. Large numbers of children in Britain, the USA and other relatively affluent countries are brought up in communities where such opportunities and facilities are well below the norms acceptable to mainstream society. Living in such conditions impacts on parenting and ultimately on the psychological and physical health of the child. Children may, therefore, suffer abuse in two ways: by poor parenting (neglect within the family) or by exclusion from societal benefits (abuse by society).

There are, in addition, other forms of oppression, identified throughout this book, which have an impact on children and contribute to child abuse.

The lack of rights of children are the most obvious of these. While great strides took place during the 1990s in relation to recognizing children's rights, as evidenced by the 1989 UN Convention on the Rights of the Child, the assertion of those rights is more problematic.

The 1989 Children Act and the 1991 *Working Together* guidelines (DoH 1991b) brought about some important improvements for children at risk of abuse – most notably their wishes and feelings must be taken into account in court hearings, reviews and conferences and in relation to decisions about placements and medicals. Children who are looked after by local authorities also now have greater rights to make representations about the quality of care they are receiving.

These are important advances which have the potential to improve the treatment of children while being investigated and assessed for risk, and also while in care. However, there are limits imposed on these developments, most notably that the child's age and understanding have to be taken into consideration when making the various decisions. While to some extent the need to place some limits on self-determination seems reasonable, there are dangers. A clear example of this lies in the scepticism that surrounds accounts by younger children about sexual abuse. Attempts to ensure that such children's evidence is more likely to be accepted by courts have proved decidedly unsuccessful (see Social Services Inspectorate 1994)

In the case of corporal punishment, the attitudes of the government and judiciary show evidence of firm resistance to furthering the rights of children. Britain and the USA lag far behind many European countries which have banned the use of physical punishment of their children by parents without, as far as is known, any adverse effects.

For many, this issue is indicative of fundamental beliefs about the nature of children and therefore of mainstream societal views about their rights. Essentially, children are seen as needing to be moulded by coercive means ('spare the rod and spoil the child') in order to be prepared for adult status and maturity.

Many child protectionists are convinced that the assertion of children's rights is a key mechanism for reducing child abuse generally. While advances have been made, they are still insufficient to have an impact on the prevention of abuse.

Related to this issue is that of oppressive attitudes towards disabled children. All too frequently there is hesitancy about investigating abuse of disabled children, particularly because of communication difficulties and beliefs that such children cannot be credible witnesses (see Marchant and Page 1992). There has been some progress in this respect in the USA by the use of what is termed assisted communication whereby those with specialist knowledge of communicating with disabled people interpret for them. However, there is still much legal wrangling over the legitimacy of such evidence.

As has been seen throughout this book, feminist ideas have had considerable impact on our thinking about and understanding of all forms of child abuse, though especially child sexual abuse. A particularly important message from this quarter is that gender socialization plays a significant part in the aetiology of child abuse and that there is, therefore, a pressing need to address this issue in child protection policy and practice. The way in which males are socialized generally, that is with the belief that strength lies in coping with one's own emotions, is dysfunctional for child care and parenting. It places more emphasis on mothers as carers, absolves males from responsibility for caring and ill equips them for it as well – physical abuse of children is sometimes a consequence. Male sexual socialization, that is with the expectation that they have stronger sexual needs than women and must be assertive and take control, helps create a climate in which child sexual abuse can happen.

These social factors have implications for front-line practice in response to child abuse referrals. Practitioners must be careful not to assume shared values, concerns and interests between parents; in particular they need to be attuned to the possibility of male violence to their partners. Further, they must make greater efforts to include men in their practice because if, as the feminist perspective argues, the roots of violence to both children and women lie in male socialization, then the logical target for change is being systematically missed (O'Hagan and Dillenberger 1995).

However, change at a broader societal level is likely to have much greater impact on preventing child abuse. There is clearly an important role for education in gender socialization, particularly in relation to sexual matters and learning to negotiate without resorting to violence.

Parental training, which is currently being considered by the government in the face of some derision, if thoughtfully applied (and universally available), may have much to commend it.

Finally, in this brief overview of broad-based preventive strategies, the issue of race and child abuse needs to be considered. While there is no evidence to suggest that black children are any more exposed to abuse than white children, they do figure more highly in care statistics (see Bebbington and Miles 1989). On the other hand, some studies have pointed to greater tentativeness about intervening in black families where there are concerns about child care (Stubbs 1989). These findings seem paradoxical. However, the explanation for the disproportionately high numbers of black children in care probably lies in the fact that black families in Britain experience higher levels of social deprivation. As regards child protection interventions, there have been some suggestions that cultural ignorance and misplaced antiracist ideas may play some part in the failure to protect black children; the Jasmine Beckford and Tyra Henry inquiries (Brent 1985; Lambeth 1987) provide clear examples of this. At the front-line level, the vital issues seem to be the need to respond sensitively and in an antiracist way to black parents without overlooking the fact that their children might be at risk and in need of protection.

At a broader level, there is need for much greater awareness of the need to tackle structures and systems that indirectly reinforce disadvantage to black people. In relation to child protection, there is a need to develop services that take into account the barriers that face black parents and children. There needs to be an awareness that many social services departments are largely controlled by white managers and geared to the needs of a white clientele. To overcome this, white professionals working with black families where abuse is suspected should be able to consult with advisers from the same cultural background as the client and should have access to interpreters where necessary. Attempts should be made to have at least one black professional at a case conference involving a black family. Chairpersons of conferences need particular awareness of an antiracist perspective and must be able to check racist assumptions in this setting. Following the adoption of measures such as these to guard against racial bias, it is important to be clear in one's mind that steps may well have to be taken to remove black children from their parents for their protection.

This type of thinking must be applied to all aspects of child protection work, not just initial investigations. Thus, therapeutic intervention and the provision of facilities such as day nurseries and family centres need to share an antiracist perspective and take as much action as possible to offset alienation of black families. Child protection work provides a particular challenge in this aspect because it is an activity that is perceived as questioning the quality of care being provided for children. It therefore generates a good deal of hostility and conflict that needs to be carefully worked through. Race and cultural issues complicate matters even further. The adoption of comprehensive and constructive antiracist policies by agencies can provide a background from which this difficult area of work can be conducted positively and with greater confidence.

It should be apparent from what has been said above that child abuse can be seen as a product of ingrained social factors such as poverty, adultism, disablism, sexism and racism. It would be simplistic to suggest that these forms of disadvantage could be easily eliminated and also that their elimination would bring an end to child abuse. Nevertheless, the linkages between factors such as these should not be underestimated, and there are two measures that could be taken immediately to begin to tackle child abuse in a more fundamentally preventive way. We could make physical punishment by parents illegal, and we could develop comprehensive training for children and young people on issues of gender, sexuality and parenting.

Developing therapeutic services for abused children and adults

The previous section has looked at what we might do to prevent child abuse. While this is clearly important in terms of the future, one of the key pressing problems of the present is how to respond to the needs of those that have already been abused. The massive extent of child abuse has only been brought home to us since the early 1980s; while it could be argued that these numbers result from broader definitions and greater sensitivity to the issue, this does not detract from what we are left with – children and adults faced with a variety of unpleasant and disabling consequences.

We are now aware that abuse of children in their own homes, on the streets and in institutions is not uncommon. We also know that some children and young people are exposed to many forms of abuse: abuse can create a vulnerability to further abuse. We also know that the experience of abuse can lead to the abuse of others. We are beginning to realize that quite large proportions of adults experiencing problems in living, such as mentally ill persons, and those who have serious drug and alcohol problems, have some history of being abused as children.

As was seen in Chapter 10, there is little in the way of a comprehensive therapeutic service available for those who have been abused or for members of their families. Child abuse has been responded to until the mid-1990s as something to be investigated and confirmed, and to be followed up in some cases with protective ongoing arrangements. Particularly in the case of physical abuse and neglect, there has been a lack of focus on the emotional needs of the child. As we have seen, the picture is different for sexual abuse. Concerns about this form of abuse were raised by those experiencing its long-term consequences; indeed this was the key catalyst for establishing it as a major social problem. However, in the 1990s, following the Cleveland inquiry, the focus was placed more on searching for evidence to prosecute the perpetrator than on the emotional needs of the abused children and their non-abusing parents.

We are not without examples of good therapeutic responses to child abuse, particularly with regard to sexual abuse. Groupwork approaches with abused girls and mothers whose children have been abused have been established in different parts of the UK. We have also seen examples of family therapeutic work. However, general studies of cases that go through the child protection system do not provide much evidence of therapeutic inputs (see Sharland *et al.* 1996; Corby 1998). The problem is that the therapeutic response is patchy and not systematic. Social workers and other child protection professionals can provide general help and support in the aftermath to an investigation, but access to more specialized psychological services seem to be a rarity.

There are other difficulties in ensuring a therapeutic response. Some children and young people may not wish initially to be involved in therapeutic services. Their early reactions to being abused may be ones of withdrawal or aggression. In some cases, the family is the key source of help and support. However, in these instances, there could be a follow-up service at a later date to see if therapeutic intervention is more appropriate at that stage, and parents could be provided with far more back-up in supporting their children, as could teachers and others having direct contact with the child.

Part of the problem is that, despite the evidence of its consequences, child abuse is not generally seen as a health issue, but much more as a social and criminal phenomenon. There is no doubt that the medical model of child abuse has considerable weaknesses in terms of providing a comprehensive account of why child abuse happens. However, in terms of understanding and responding to its effects, there seems to be a major health component to child abuse and its consequences and a gaping hole waiting to be filled (see Oates 1996).

Responding to offenders

In contrast to the lack of development of therapeutic services, there has been a considerable rise in interest in the 1990s in dealing with child abuse offenders. The main focus has been on sex offenders or paedophiles who became the bogeymen of the late twentieth century. The main model of the paedophile is someone who abuses children outside the family, gaining access to children in public places, youth clubs, day centres and residential settings. He is seen as unequivocally dangerous and as a criminal. The appropriate response to such individuals has been seen to identify them and ensure that children are protected from them.

There have been several important and protective measures that have been put into place to tackle the paedophile problem. First, there have been changes in legal procedures to ensure that child witnesses are better able to give evidence in criminal trials. Second, there have been greater efforts to work with sex offenders in prison and while on probation using cognitive methods to try and reduce the likelihood of further offending. Third, there have been developments in tracking sex offenders after release from prison; they are required to lodge their addresses with the police and notify them of housing moves. Fourth, they are required to be registered so that they can be identified should they seek employment which gives them access to children.

Many of these measures seem eminently sensible. While there has been an element of hysteria about paedophiles, with local newspapers reporting their addresses and community protests being made in order to move them on, the concerns of parents about risks to their children, though not statistically supported, are understandable.

However, there are some dysfunctions in this process, particularly in relation to intrafamilial child sexual abuse. First, the emphasis on the dangerous extrafamilial paedophile can draw attention away from intrafamilial abuse. Second, where intrafamilial abuse is discovered, it can lead to particularly punitive responses as a result of all those that sexually abuse children being seen in the same light as the worst offenders. Such an interpretation may not fit all abusers by any means, and there is some evidence to suggest that we need to keep a more open mind in relation to some (though not automatically all) intrafamilial abusers. A key problem resulting from this way of thinking is the adoption of defensive practices which while ensuring the protection of the child at one level may leave all sorts of problems and difficulties at another. The practice of removing males from households is one example of this. While this is a sensible measure at the more extreme end of the abuse spectrum, it is important to ensure that it does not become an automatic measure. Similarly, the trend to criminalize all child abusive behaviour can have dysfunctions in terms of providing support and treatment for both those who have been abused and for abusers. The threat of criminalization usually leads to silence on the part of abusers, so they cannot be helped. Some children abused within the family do not wish their abusers to be prosecuted; as a result they may be deterred from divulging what has happened to them.

Child sexual abuse within the family seems to take so many forms that one-dimensional responses are inadequate (see Corby 1998). It is clear that the criminal law must provide a backdrop to child protection work, but the impact of criminalization on working therapeutically and supportively with children, mothers and fathers must be taken into account. As we have seen from examples in the Netherlands, Belgium and the USA, it is possible with flexibility to use the criminal law more positively to enforce therapeutic intervention.

Concluding comments

It will be clear from the research and ideas reviewed in this book that the notion of child abuse is a shifting and much-contested one. It may even be a term that is starting to outlive its usefulness. For some it is a term that has too negative connotations as we shift towards trying to work more supportively with families to overcome problems that contribute to their children's diswelfare. For others, however, it is a term that ensures that the need for child protection is not over-looked in our efforts to improve family situations.

Whatever term we use, the need for a governmental strategy to ensure that children's needs for their proper growth and development are met is obvious. This is not an easy task, and the ebbs and flows of policy in the second half of the twentieth century were testimony to this. However, the knowledge we now have about the ill consequences and costs of the various forms of child mistreatment, both to individuals and society, demands a concerted approach at levels over and beyond those that characterized the 1980s and 1990s, that is reactive and often poorly funded efforts to identify and police individual cases.

Above all, there is a need for concerted preventive measures at a broader societal level and for a proper system for responding to the psychological needs of all involved in child abuse situations.

NOTES

Chapter 2   Childhood, child abuse and history

1 There are some British histories of social work. Younghusband (1978) deals with the period from 1950 to 1975. Yelloly (1980) looks at the influence of psychoanalysis on social work practice from the 1930s onwards. The most comprehensive studies are those by Woodroofe (1962) and Seed (1973).

2   This day a quarter past two in the afternoone my Mary fell asleepe in the Lord, her soule past into that rest where the body of Jesus, and the soules of the saints are, shee was: 8 yeares and 45 days old when shee dyed, my soule had aboundant cause to blesse god for her, who was our first fruites, and those god would have offered to him, and this I freely resigned up to him[,] it was a pretious child, a bundle of myrrhe, a bundle of sweetnes, shee was a child of ten thousand, full of wisedome, woman-like gravity, knowledge, sweet expressions of god, apt in her learning, tender hearted and loving, an obedient child [to us.] it was free from [the rudenesse of] litle children, it was to us as a boxe of sweet ointment, which now its broken smells more deliciously than it did before, Lord I rejoyce I had such a present for thee, it was patient in the sicknesse, thankefull to admiracion; it lived desired and dyed lamented, thy memory is and wille bee sweete unto mee. [26 May 1650]

(Macfarlane 1970: 203)

3 It should be noted that Boswell (1990) has been criticized by some historians for being over-optimistic about the fate of abandoned children (see Tilly *et al.* 1992).

4 This statement, while demonstrating public concern about child sexual abuse, also shows that there was probably a hierarchy of concerns. No mention is made of female children and those of non-citizen status.

5 La Fontaine (1990: 210), drawing from anthropological work, lends some support to such a view with regard to sexual abuse.

Chapter 3   A history of child abuse and neglect 1870–1991

1 It would be wrong, however, to suggest that there was no relevant legislation at all. The 1868 Poor Law Act made wilful neglect by a parent of a child under 14 that threatened or resulted in serious injury and offence. The weakness of this law was that only Poor Law officials were empowered to bring cases of this kind to court and they very rarely did so. The 1861 Offences Against the Person Act could also be used to prosecute parents for assaults on their children, but no particular agency was mandated to report or seek out such abuse.

2 The major legislative change of this period was the 1933 Children and Young Persons Act, which followed in the tradition of previous legislation by extending the range of prosecutable offences against children. It also blurred distinctions between neglected children and young offenders by such measures as the creation of approved schools for all who came into these two categories (before this they had attended separate institutions). By 1946, when the Curtis Committee reported, this type of thinking was well established: 'According to the evidence of the Home Office, it is often an accident whether a child is before the court for an offence or as a neglected child, and it is accordingly appropriate that the same methods of treatment be equally available' (para. 38, p. 14).

3 See Housden (1955: 209–10), which provides an extract of an NSPCC inspector's discovery of and response to a child sexual abuse case. The case is undated, but as the children involved were committed to industrial schools, it must have been before the implementation of the 1933 Children and Young Persons Act. The case involved a 12-year-old girl, her 11-year-old sister and her 9-year-old brother. Their mother was dead and they were living with their father and a 46-year-old male lodger. It was revealed that the two girls slept in the same bed as the lodger. The inspector's records described the children as being dirty and neglected. A medical examination was arranged by the inspector. 'This proved that the girl aged 12 had been interfered with.' The father and the lodger were prosecuted. The father, a first-time offender, received a light sentence and the lodger 18 months' hard labour. The children, as mentioned above, were committed to industrial schools. The tenor of the report is very factual. The response to this case comes across as insensitive by our standards but unequivocally child protective.

4 See Cleveland inquiry report (Butler-Sloss 1988: para. 4.80, p. 64). A 10-year-old girl and her two siblings were examined with their mother's consent by Dr Higgs in the hospital. Their father removed them. They were subsequently brought into police custody under place of safety orders and examined by a police surgeon, Dr Beeby. His diagnosis conflicted with that of Dr Higgs, who re-examined the children. The following day they were re-examined by Dr Irvine, another police surgeon. The report adds that the children 'were later examined by three more doctors'.

Chapter 4   Child protection and family support in the 1990s

1 La Fontaine (1998: 9–12) provided some useful information about the different terminologies used to describe this form of abuse. The term 'Satanic'

implies that children are being abused as part of devil-worship ceremonies, and is usually by Christians of an extreme fundamentalist nature who are committed to wiping out such forms of worship. The term 'Satanist' is used by those who attribute the abuse to devil-worship, but do not believe in the devil; their concerns are more objectively focused on child abuse issues. 'Ritual abuse' is a term used to describe any form of child abuse taking place within a ritual setting (including devil-worship).

2 The accounts of the interviews with the child, MT, are a very good example of this (see Clyde 1992: paras 11.91–11.96). MT is described in the report as an 'articulate and able child who rarely showed visible signs of emotion. She appeared very grown up' (para. 11.91). In the following paragraphs she gives a clear and detailed account of taking part in a ritual where children were hurt 'in the wrong places'.

3 Jason Swift was a 14-year-old boy at the time of his death in 1985. He was living on the streets and had been doing sexual acts for money for some time. He was drugged and slowly suffocated to death while being sexually abused by four men, who were later convicted of manslaughter. They were given sentences of between $13\frac{1}{2}$ years' and 19 years' imprisonment.

4 Part 8 Reviews were introduced in 1991 in the *Working Together* guidelines (DoH 1991b). Such reviews are required to be carried out by area child protection committees where child abuse has taken place resulting in death or serious injury likely to be of major public concern. The reports resulting from the reviews must be sent to the Department of Health and the findings must be considered by the relevant agencies within the area where the abuse has taken place. A key aim of this review system is to ensure that lessons are learned and put into practice as soon as possible.

Chapter 5 Defining child abuse

1 Stephanie Fox was known by the health and welfare authorities to have suffered minor bruising on 30 occasions before she died as a result of a violent assault by her father. They had previously declined to remove Stephanie, probably because their expectations of the family were very low and it was felt that such bruising (largely perceived to be the result of careless supervision of the child rather than of physical mistreatment) was not remarkable given the background of the Fox family. The Lester Chapman case shows a similarly resigned acceptance of low standards of care, as does that of the case of Paul. In the case of Tyra Henry, the social worker made assumptions about Caribbean culture that placed heavy expectations on this child's grandmother to provide care and protection for her. West Indian grandmothers were stereotypically considered to be the linch-pins of the family as far as child care was concerned. As far as Beatrice Henry was concerned, nothing could have been further from the truth. She had experienced the death of her husband and the severe mistreatment of her grandson. She was a lone parent dealing with the problems of her own three children, was inadequately housed and had multiple debts. As events proved, she was completely unable to protect Tyra.

2 The following two vignettes, with consequences in parentheses, are taken from Giovannoni and Becerra's (1979: 116) study and give a flavour of the general approach used: 'The parents regularly left their child alone outside the house during the day until almost dark (neighbours have spotted the child wandering five blocks from home).' 'The parents banged the child against the wall while shaking him by the shoulders (the child suffered a concussion)' (Giovannoni and Becerra 1979: 113).

3 Section 31(2) of the 1989 Children Act states:

> A court may only make a care order or supervision order if it is satisfied –
>
> (a) that the child concerned is suffering, or is likely to suffer, significant harm; and
> (b) that the harm, or likelihood of harm, is attributable to –
> > (i) the care given to the child, or likely to be given to him if the order were not made, not being what it would be reasonable to expect a parent to give to him; or
> > (ii) the child's being beyond parental control.

Section 31(9) states: '"harm" means ill-treatment or the impairment of health or development; "development" means physical, intellectual, emotional, social or behavioural development; "ill-treatment" includes sexual abuse and forms of ill-treatment which are not physical'.

4 See Baldwin and Oliver (1975), Smith (1975) and Greenland (1987). However, these are all retrospective studies. Although the vast majority of the severely ill-treated children they studied had had minor bruising at an earlier date, this does not mean that all children with minor bruising will be severely abused in the future.

5 Issues of this kind were highlighted in the Doreen Aston report (Lambeth, Lewisham and Southwark 1989). Before Doreen's birth, her mother Christine Mason had had a child, Karl, who died aged 10 weeks. A postmortem revealed that he had three fractured ribs and a subdural haemorrhage, but these injuries were not thought to have contributed to his death, which was finally recorded as a cot death (see Lambeth, Lewisham and Southwark 1989: paras 11 and 12, p. 8). The authors of the report felt that the cot death decision led social workers and others to overlook the fact that the child had been abused and, therefore, that subsequent children might be particularly at risk.

6 Political factors may also play a part in this relative lack of urgency. Wolock and Horowitz (1984) argued that neglect of children is far more common than physical abuse in the USA, but receives far less attention. This 'neglect of neglect', as they termed it, results from the fact that closer inspection of many children's lives would reveal the extent to which poverty contributes to neglect and this would create political embarrassments for governments.

7 Brent (1985: 69–74) provided useful detailed material on the failure-to-thrive syndrome. At birth, Jasmine weighed 5 lb. 11 oz. By 4 months, she had reached an average weight for a child of her age and, therefore, would have been expected to maintain this average growth throughout her early childhood. After 10 months, Jasmine had slipped back and her weight was well below the average. It was below the third centile (that is Jasmine was among

the 3 per cent most poorly developed of all children). At age 15 months Jasmine weighed 18 lb. 6 oz., even further down in the third centile. At 20 months, when she experienced her first serious injury, she was still well down in the third centile. At the age of 27 months, after she had been in foster care for seven months, Jasmine had grown considerably and weighed 25 lb. 5 oz. (on the 25th centile). At this point she was returned to her mother and step-father. She was not weighed again until her death 27 months later. She weighed 23 lb.

Chapter 6   The extent of child abuse

1 It is important to distinguish between the terms 'prevalence' and 'incidence'. Prevalence studies measure how many people in a given sample have experienced a particular phenomenon at least once over a particular period of time. Incidence studies measure the number of occurrences of a particular phenomenon in a given sample of people over a particular period of time. Thus, if a sample of 100 people were asked if they had been sexually abused at least once before the age of 15, and 20 said that they had, the prevalence rate of abuse of such children would be 20 per cent. If these 100 people were asked how often they had been sexually abused before the age of 15, the answer would probably be higher. They might report abuse on 60 occasions. The incidence rate of abuse would then be 60 per 100 people over the first 15 years of their lives. La Fontaine (1990: ch. 2) gives a fuller, very useful account of these and other issues relating to prevalence and incidence studies.

2 Those families with just 1- and 2-year-old children were omitted because one of the study's objectives was to measure sibling violence. How this affects the interpretation of the findings (that is are they an underestimate or overestimate of the total) is unclear. It is worth noting, however, that in 1998–9, the registration rate for children physically abused in the first year of their lives in England was much higher than for all the other age groupings.

Chapter 7   Who abuses whom

1 In the case of Wayne Brewer, who was killed by his stepfather, Nigel Briffett, his mother was heavily implicated. In a report written for court when Wayne was made the subject of a care order, the social worker commented on her as follows: 'Her inability to restrain her husband, together with the rather negative handling of the child, characterised by her unwillingness to readily handle him, and to generally care for and stimulate him, indicate that she has not really been able to accept responsibility for him' (Somerset Area Review Committee 1977).

2 The views put forward on this subject in the Cleveland report are of interest. The term 'collusive mother' is not explicitly used. However, the implications are clear.

Again quoting Professor Sir Martin Roth, 'In many cases mothers play a role in the genesis of the sexual abuse of their daughters. They may be too physically ill or inadequate in personality to provide proper care and protection for their children. In other cases mothers elect the eldest or one of the oldest daughters to the role of "child mother". The girl in her early teens or even earlier is expected to take the responsibility for the caring of the younger children whose mothering role is allowed to slide into a sexual relationship with the father. This is tolerated with little or no protest. I refer to lack of protest of [sic] the part of the mother for a variety of reasons and the mother may in such cases deny what is happening. She conceals the truth from herself as well as others; the relationship continues and when the situation is brought to light it may be insisted by the mother that it had been unknown to her.'

(Butler-Sloss 1988: para. 29, p. 8)

3 That women do physically abuse children is not being denied. For an interesting case study of women who have fatally abused their children see Korbin (1989).

4 We need to be sceptical about making sweeping distinctions between extrafamilial and intrafamilial child sexual abusers. It may well be that overall, Groth and Burgess's (1979) abusers were more serious abusers and more traumatized as children than those seen by Ben-Tovim *et al.* (1988) and that there are, therefore, some overall differences between those who abuse outside and within the family. However, because of our lack of knowledge about intrafamilial abusers, we need to be careful in drawing conclusions. There seems to be a wide spectrum of types of intrafamilial sexual abuse ranging from persistent gross abuse to single incidents of a less serious nature at the time of discovery (see Corby 1998). It would be interesting to know whether more serious intrafamilial abusers had been more exposed to abuse themselves as children than those involved in more isolated, less serious incidents.

5 In 1996, 33 per cent of all live births in England and Wales were outside marriage, though for 80 per cent of these births there was joint registration. In 1996 lone-parent families constituted 21 per cent of all families with dependent children in Great Britain. This is three times the percentage in 1971, but it is worth noting that in the 1990s there was no increase. Britain has the second highest divorce rate among countries in the European Union – in 1995 divorces involved 161,000 children under the age of 16, twice as many as in 1971. In 1991, there were half a million step-families in Britain involving a million children (both birth-children and stepchildren).

6 Christine Mason, the mother of Doreen Aston, was known to have been depressed in October 1985, seven months before Doreen was born. In January 1985, her 10-week-old son, Karl, had died in suspicious circumstances (see Chapter 4: n. 8). Nine months later Christine was said to be continuing 'to give cause for concern as she was carrying the ashes of her dead child around with her' (Lambeth, Lewisham and Southwark 1989: ch. 2, para. 15, p. 9). There is no further reference to depression or grief reaction in the report.

Beatrice Henry, Tyra Henry's grandmother, on whom great reliance was placed by Lambeth Social Services Department for her protection, had experienced the death of her husband and the maiming and loss of her grandson in 1982 (she had also previously suffered the death of her own son). The inquiry report points out that there was 'not a line in the contemporary records and not a line in the evidence given to us which recognises that by the time of Tyra's birth, Beatrice Henry was struggling with private grief along with the difficulties of her daily life' (Lambeth 1987: 112). The inquiry panel recommended that social workers receive training in this area and be directed to devote attention to such matters in future.

The Koseda inquiry noted that the cohabitation of Heidi Koseda's mother, Rosemary, with Nicholas Price 'seems to have been the start of a marked deterioration in her mental state and way of life, which culminated in serious mental illness after the discovery of Heidi's body early in 1985' (Hillingdon 1986: para. 1.1).

7 In the cases of Tyra Henry (Lambeth 1987) and Darryn Clarke (DHSS 1979) there do not seem to have been obvious signs of conflict. However, very little information seems to come to light about the relationships of parents or parent substitutes in public inquiry reports. Both Andrew Neil and Charles Courtney, who were convicted for the killing of these children, had histories of violence. The lack of conflict in their relationships with these children's mothers may have been the result of their being totally dominating and controlling figures.

8 Doreen Aston, Stephanie Fox and Tyra Henry and their families were all under financial and material stress at the times of their births and in their early childhoods. This was particularly apparent in the case of Stephanie Fox. The Fox family, consisting of mother, father, Stephanie (aged 2), and twins (aged 8 months), were eventually provided with accommodation on the 19th floor of a tower block. They suffered chronic financial problems, despite help being given by social workers under section 1 of the 1980 Child Care Act. The report, while acknowledging this help, comments: 'Despite the desperate circumstances of families in [a] crisis of this kind, we believe that section 1 financial help should be used whenever possible as part of a consistent plan to promote the well-being of children in families, rather than as a routine response to crisis calls for help' (Wandsworth 1990: 72).

9 Stephen Menheniott was $19\frac{1}{2}$ years old when he died as a result of multiple injuries inflicted on him over a long period of time by his father. Because of his age, this case could be seen to be the murder of a young adult, but this judgement would belie the true nature of Stephen's abuse. The events of his life and death all carry the hallmarks of a case of child abuse. His father, Thomas Menheniott, was brought up in public care institutions. Nearly all his eight children had had long spells in care. He had convictions for neglect and ill-treatment of his children and had been acquitted after being charged with incest. Stephen was a rather pathetic, immature young man. He had spent the bulk of his life in residential care attending schools for maladjusted children and had developed few lasting relationships. He was returned to his father's 'care' at the age of $15\frac{1}{2}$. He was clearly exposed to prolonged physical abuse and intimidation.

Chapter 8   The causation of child abuse

1 Sociobiology emerged as an identifiable discipline in the 1970s (Wilson 1975). It is essentially a new form of social Darwinism, but is more subtly

argued than its predecessor. Sociobiologists' main proposition is that social sciences have been too narrow in their interpretations of human behaviour, associating it almost exclusively with cultural and social influences. In this process, the fact that humans are, like any other form of living species, biologically driven, has been forgotten. From a sociobiological perspective, biological forces, particularly gene preservation, are paramount influences on behaviour (Dawkins 1976). Social scientists have responded by arguing that sociobiology has theoretical flaws and adverse political effects, such as the potential for encouraging racism, sexism and far right views such as eugenics (Sahlins 1977; Montagu 1980). In many ways, this conflict is part of the continuing nature–nurture debate which has existed formally since the emergence of the social sciences in the eighteenth century.

2 For a mainstream analysis see Stafford-Clark (1965), Fancher (1973) and Jahoda (1977). Kline (1981) provided details of empirical studies into Freudian theory. Feminist critiques of Freudian theory are to be found in Mitchell (1974: 61–108) and Sydie (1987: 125–67).

3 Steele and Pollock (1974: 128–30), in discussing the non-abusing parent, pointed out that 'The other parent almost invariably contributes, however, to the abusive behaviour either by openly accepting it or by more subtly abetting it, consciously or unconsciously.' They listed various forms in which this happens, one of which seems to have been apparent in several of the inquiry report cases in Britain, for example Darryn Clarke (DHSS 1979), Jasmine Beckford (Brent 1985) and Kimberley Carlile (Greenwich 1987): 'One parent feeling overwhelmed and frustrated may turn the infant over to the other with admonitions to do something more drastic to stop the baby's annoying behaviour.' How voluntary such behaviour is, is open to question. The non-abusing parent may be forced to hand over the child for such inappropriate discipline. With regard to the contribution of children to their own abuse Steele and Pollock (1974) stressed that 'characteristics presented by the infant, such as sex, time of birth, health status, and behavior are factors in instigating child abuse'.

4 Steele and Pollock's (1974) views on the influence of socio-economic factors on the incidence of child abuse are that they are marginal:

> Basically they are irrelevant to the actual act of child beating. Unquestionably, social and economic difficulties and disasters put added stress on people's lives and contribute to behavior which might otherwise remain dormant. But such factors must be considered as incidental enhancers rather than necessary and sufficient causes.
>
> (Steele and Pollock 1974: 108)

5 Smith (1991) outlines the parts of the 1989 Children Act that specifically enhance a children's rights perspective. Two examples are, first, section 22, which emphasizes the need to consult children of sufficient age and understanding with regard to all decisions that affect them (this section is very similar to section 18 of the 1980 Child Care Act) and, second, section 44(7), which gives a child of sufficient age and understanding the right to refuse a medical examination under an emergency protection order (a direct result of events in Cleveland, where it was felt that children were exposed to many assessments and examinations without having any recourse if they objected). In general, the 1989 Children Act was a move towards greater

consideration of children as subjects rather than objects. However, the legislation still leaves a lot of room for adultist views to prevail.

Chapter 9   The consequences of child abuse

1 Jasmine Beckford's stepfather, Morris, spent the first nine years of his life with his grandmother in Jamaica before being reunited with his parents in Britain. At age 13, he and his sister were severely beaten by both parents and forced to sleep in an outhouse with no bed and one blanket between them before being taken into care (Brent 1985: 42). It is not known how Tyra Henry's father, Andrew Neil, was treated as a child. His mother left home when he was aged 7. He was noted to have hysterical fits at age 10 and physically assaulted a 2-year-old baby when he was aged 13 (Lambeth 1987: 8–10). Unfortunately, not enough is known about the background of fathers in many other public inquiry cases for a variety of reasons. Closer attention to their biographical details (and those of the mothers) would undoubtedly add to our understanding of the causes of such gross violence to children.

2 Carmen et al. (1984) show considerable awareness of the potential impact of physical and sexual abuse on women:

> In our sample, the abused females directed their hatred and aggression against themselves in both overt and covert ways. These behaviours formed a continuum from quiet resignation and depression to repeated episodes of self-mutilation and suicide attempts . . . Markedly impaired self-esteem was prominent among these patients, as they conveyed a sense that they were undeserving of any empathic understanding or help by clinicians.
>
> (Carmen et al. 1984: 382)

These reactions were in contrast to the outwardly directed aggression that was most common among the mentally ill males in this study with a history of abuse. From this perspective, the form of the reaction to abuse is heavily influenced by social and socialization factors. Similarly, being black and abused in predominantly white-dominated societies also influences the consequences and the response to the abuse (see Angelou 1984).

3 Gordon (1989) points out that some of what have been termed 'negative' effects of child sexual abuse, such as running away and inappropriate sexual behaviour, could be seen as positive reactions to the situations many of the girls in the records she studied were faced with. ' "Sex delinquency" was an escape route not only of victims, but often of highly responsible victims, trying to avoid telling their secrets and exploding their families' (Gordon 1989: 240).

Chapter 10   Research into child protection practice

1 Darryn Clarke was never seen by social workers before his death. The focus of the inquiry was on the response to the initial allegation and the reasons for the delay in tracing a child who was said to be at risk. Similarly, Kimberley

Carlile was not known to the social services department to whom allegations of ill-treatment were made. However, in this case there had been prior social work involvement by other social services departments. The inquiry concentrated on the delays and difficulties associated with assessing whether Kimberley was at risk or not.

2 Parents Anonymous groups were first set up in California in 1969 (see Holmes 1978). Small voluntary groups of parents who have abused their children meet a professional group helper to share and discuss feelings and issues. The aim is to help such parents improve their self-image and provide support for each other. Parents are encouraged to contact each other regularly outside the group and to follow up parents who drop out. There is no direct equivalent in Britain. Organizations such as Parents Against Injustice and the Family Rights Group are pressure groups organized to challenge the child protection system.

Chapter 11 Current issues in child protection work

1 Another category of abused children that could be included here is that of children living in war zones (see Elbedour *et al.* 1993).

BIBLIOGRAPHY

Abel, G., Mittelman, M. and Becker, J. (1985) Sexual offenders: results of assessment and recommendations for treatment, in H. Ben-Aron, S. Hucker, and C. Webster (eds) *Clinical Criminology*. Toronto: M. M. Graphics.

Abel, G., Becker, J., Mittelman, M. *et al.* (1987) Self-reported sex crimes of nonincarcerated paraphiliacs, *Journal of Interpersonal Violence*, 2: 3–25.

Adams, J., McLellan, J., Douglass, D., McCurry, C. and Storck, M. (1995) Sexually inappropriate behaviours in seriously mentally ill children and adolescents, *Child Abuse and Neglect*, 19: 555–68.

Adams-Tucker, C. (1981) A socioclinical overview of 28 sex-abused children, *Child Abuse and Neglect*, 5: 361–7.

Adler, N. and Schutz, J. (1995) Sibling incest offenders, *Child Abuse and Neglect*, 19: 811–19.

Allen, A. and Morton, A. (1961) *This is Your Child: The Story of the NSPCC*. London: Routledge & Kegan Paul.

Allen, R. and Oliver, J. (1982) The effects of child maltreatment on language development, *Child Abuse and Neglect*, 6: 299–305.

Ammerman, R., von Hasselt, V., Hersen, M., McConigle, J. and Lubetsky, M. (1989) Abuse and neglect in psychiatrically hospitalised multi-handicapped children, *Child Abuse and Neglect*, 13: 335–43.

Anderson, S., Bach, C. and Griffin, S. (1981) Psychosocial sequelae in intra-familial victims of sexual assault and abuse. Paper presented at the Third International Congress on Child Abuse and Neglect, Amsterdam.

Angelou, M. (1983) *I Know Why the Caged Bird Sings*. London: Virago.

Argles, P. (1980) Attachment and child abuse, *British Journal of Social Work*, 10: 33–42.

Ariès, P. (1962) *Centuries of Childhood*. Harmondsworth: Penguin.

Armstrong, L. (1978) *Kiss Daddy Goodnight*. New York: Dell.

Asen, K., George, E., Piper, R. and Stevens, A. (1989) A systems approach to child abuse: management and treatment issues, *Child Abuse and Neglect*, 13: 45–57.

Association of Chief Officers of Probation (ACOP) (1996) *Sex Offenders Survey*. London: ACOP.

Association of the Directors of Social Services (ADSS) (1988) Press release, July.

Audit Commission (1994) *Seen but not Heard: Coordinating Community Child Health and Social Services for Children in Need*. London: HMSO.

Augoustinos, M. (1987) Developmental effects of child abuse, *Child Abuse and Neglect*, 11: 15–27.

Badinter, E. (1981) *The Myth of Motherhood: An Historical View of the Maternal Instinct*. New York: Macmillan.

Bagley, C. and Ramsay, R. (1986) Sexual abuse in childhood: psychosocial outcomes and implications for social work practice, *Journal of Social Work and Human Sexuality*, 4: 33–47.

Baher, E., Hyman, C., Jones, C., Kerr, A. and Mitchell, R. (1976) *At Risk: An Account of the Battered Child Research Department*. London: Routledge and Kegan Paul.

Baker, A. and Duncan, S. (1985) Child sexual abuse: a study of prevalence in Great Britain, *Child Abuse and Neglect*, 9: 457–67.

Baldwin, J. and Oliver, J. (1975) Epidemiology and family characteristics of severely abused children, *British Journal of Social and Preventive Medicine*, 29: 205–21.

Bandura, A. (1965) *Principles of Behaviour Modification*. New York: Holt, Rinehart and Winston.

Banning, A. (1989) Mother–son incest: confronting a prejudice, *Child Abuse and Neglect*, 13: 563–70.

Barash, D. (1981) *Sociobiology: The Whisperings Within*. London: Fontana.

Barnardo's (1998) *Whose Daughter Next? Children Abused Through Prostitution*. London: Barnardo's.

Barratt, A., Trepper, T. and Fish, L. (1990) Feminist informed family therapy for the treatment of intra-familial child sexual abuse, *Journal of Family Psychology*, 4: 151–66.

Bebbington, A. and Miles, J. (1989) The background of children who enter local authority care, *British Journal of Social Work*, 19: 349–68.

Beck, U. (1992) *Risk Society: Towards a New Modernity*. London: Sage.

Becker, J. and Quinsey, V. (1993) Assessing suspected child molesters, *Child Abuse and Neglect*, 17: 169–74.

Becker, S. and Macpherson, S. (eds) (1988) *Public Issues, Private Pain: Poverty, Social Work and Social Policy*. London: Social Services Insight Books.

Behlmer, G. (1982) *Child Abuse and Moral Reform in England 1870–1908*. Stanford, CA: Stanford University Press.

Beitchman, J., Zucker, K., Hood, J., Da Costa, G. and Akman, D. (1991) A review of the short-term effects of child sexual abuse, *Child Abuse and Neglect*, 15: 537–56.

Beitchman, J., Zucker, K., Hood, J. *et al.* (1992) A review of the long-term effects of child sexual abuse, *Child Abuse and Neglect*, 16: 101–18.

Belsky, J. (1980) Child maltreatment: an ecological integration, *American Psychologist*, 35: 320–35.

Belsky, J. and Vondra, J. (1989) Lessons from child abuse: the determinants of parenting, in D. Cicchetti and V. Carlson (eds) *Child Maltreatment: Theory and Research on the Causes and Consequences of Child Abuse and Neglect*. Cambridge: Cambridge University Press.

Benedict, M. and White, R. (1985) Selected perinatal factors and child abuse, *American Journal of Public Health*, 75: 780–1.

Benedict, M., White, R., Wulff, L. and Hall, B. (1990) Reported maltreatment in children with multiple disabilities, *Child Abuse and Neglect*, 14: 207–17.

Ben-Tovim, A., Elton, A., Hildebrand, J., Tranter, M. and Vizard, E. (eds) (1988) *Child Sexual Abuse Within the Family: Assessment and Treatment: The Work of the Great Ormond Street Team*. London: Wright.

Bergner, R., Delgado, L. and Graybill, D. (1994) Finkelhor's risk factor checklist: a cross-validation study, *Child Abuse and Neglect*, 18: 331–40.

Berkshire (County Council) (1979) *Lester Chapman Inquiry Report*. Reading: Berkshire County Council.

Berliner, L. and Conte, R. (1995) The effects of disclosure and intervention on sexually abused children, *Child Abuse and Neglect*, 19: 371–84.

Besharov, D. (1981) Towards better research on child abuse and neglect: making definitional issues an explicit methodological concern, *Child Abuse and Neglect*, 5: 383–90.

Bibby, P. (ed.) (1996) *Organised Abuse: The Current Debate*. Aldershot: Aldgate.

Biehal, N., Clayden, J., Stein, M. and Wade, J. (1995) *Moving On: Young People and Leaving Care Schemes*. London: HMSO.

Birchall, E. (1989) The frequency of child abuse: what do we really know?, in O. Stevenson (ed.) *Child Abuse: Public Policy and Professional Practice*. Hemel Hempstead: Harvester-Wheatsheaf.

Birchall, E. with Hallett, C. (1995) *Working Together in Child Protection*. London: HMSO.

Bools, C., Neale, B. and Meadow, R. (1994) Munchausen Syndrome by Proxy: a study of psychopathology, *Child Abuse and Neglect*, 18: 773–88.

Boswell, J. (1990) *The Kindness of Strangers: The Abandonment of Children in Western Europe from Late Antiquity to the Renaissance*. New York: Vintage.

Bourn, D. (1993) Over-chastisement, child compliance and parenting skills: a behavioural intervention by a family centre worker, *British Journal of Social Work*, 23: 481–99.

Bowlby, J. (1951) *Maternal Care and Mental Health: A Report Prepared on Behalf of the World Health Organization as a Contribution to the United Nations Programme for the Welfare of Homeless Children*. Geneva: World Health Organization.

Bowlby, J. (1971) *Attachment and Loss: Volume 1, Attachment*. Harmondsworth: Penguin.

Bowlby, J., Fry, S. and Ainsworth, M. (1965) *Child Care and the Growth of Love*. Harmondsworth: Penguin.

Brady, K. (1979) *Father's Days: A True Story of Incest*. New York: Dell.

Brekke, J. (1987) Detecting wife and child abuse in clinical settings, *Social Casework*, 68: 332–8.

Brent (London Borough of) (1985) *A Child in Trust: The Report of the Panel of Inquiry into the Circumstances Surrounding the Death of Jasmine Beckford*. London: London Borough of Brent.

Brewster, A., Nelson, J., Hymel, K., *et al.* (1998) Victim, perpetrator, family and incident characteristics of 32 infant maltreatment deaths in the United States Air Force, *Child Abuse and Neglect*, 22: 91–101.

Bridge (Child Care Consultancy Service) (1991) *Sukina: An Evaluation of the Circumstances Leading to her Death*. London: The Bridge.

Bridge (Child Care Consultancy Service) (1995a) *Paul: Death from Neglect*. London: The Bridge.

Bridge (Child Care Consultancy Service) (1995b) *Overview Report in Respect of Charmaine and Heather West*. Gloucester: Gloucestershire Area Child Protection Committee.

Bridge (Child Care Consultancy Service) (1997) *Risk Assessment Schedule, Version 2*, March. London: The Bridge.

Bridge (Child Care Consultancy Service) (1998) *Dangerous Care: Working to Protect Children*. London: The Bridge.

Briere, J. (1984) The long-term effects of childhood sexual abuse: defining a post-sexual-abuse syndrome. Paper presented at the Third National Conference on the Sexual Victimization of Children, Washington, DC.

Briggs, L. and Joyce, P. (1997) What determines post-traumatic stress disorder symptomatology for survivors of child sexual abuse, *Child Abuse and Neglect*, 21: 575–82.

Bristow, E. (1977) *Vice and Vigilance*. Dublin: Gill and Macmillan.

Brown, C. (1984) *Black and White Britain: The Third PSI Survey*. London: Heinemann.

Brown, C. (1986) *Child Abuse Parents Speaking: Parents' Impressions of Social Workers and the Social Work Process*, working paper. Bristol: Bristol School of Applied and Urban Studies.

Brown, G. and Harris, T. (1978) *Social Origins of Depression: A Study of Psychiatric Disorder in Women*. London: Tavistock.

Brown, T. and Waters, J. (1985) *Parental Participation at Case Conferences*. Rochdale: BASPCAN (British Association for the Prevention of Cruelty and Neglect).

Browne, A. and Finkelhor, D. (1986) Initial and long-term effects: a review of the research, in D. Finkelhor *et al.* (eds) *A Sourcebook on Child Sexual Abuse*. Beverly Hills, CA: Sage.

Browne, K. and Herbert, M. (1997) *Preventing Family Violence*. Chichester: Wiley.

Browne, K. and Saqi, S. (1988) Approaches to screening for child abuse and neglect, in K. Browne, C. Davies and P. Stratton (eds) *Early Prediction and Prevention of Child Abuse*. Chichester: Wiley.

Burgdorff, K. (1981) *Recognition of and Reporting of Child Maltreatment from the National Study of Incidence and Severity of Child Abuse and Neglect*. Washington, DC: National Center on Child Abuse and Neglect.

Burnett, B. (1993) The psychological abuse of latency age children: a survey, *Child Abuse and Neglect*, 17: 441–54.

Burton, D., Nesmith, A. and Badten, L. (1997) Clinicians' views on sexually aggressive children and their families, *Child Abuse and Neglect*, 21: 157–70.

Butler-Sloss, Lord Justice E. (1988) *Report of the Inquiry into Child Abuse in Cleveland 1987*, Cmnd 412. London: HMSO.

Calam, R. and Franchi, C. (1987) *Child Abuse and its Consequences*. Cambridge: Cambridge University Press.

Calam, R., Horn, L., Glasgow, D. and Cox, A. (1998) Psychological disturbance and child sexual abuse: a follow-up study, *Child Abuse and Neglect*, 22: 901–13.

Campbell, B. (1988) *Unofficial Secrets*. London: Virago.

Campbell, M. (1991) Children at risk: how different are children on child abuse registers?, *British Journal of Social Work*, 21: 259–75.

Camras, L. and Rappaport, S. (1993) Conflict behaviors of maltreated and non-maltreated children, *Child Abuse and Neglect*, 17: 455–64.

Carmen, E., Rieker, P. and Mills, T. (1984) Victims of violence and psychiatric illness, *American Journal of Psychiatry*, 141: 378–83.

Carty, H. (1988) Brittle or battered?, *Archives of Disease in Childhood*, 63: 350–2.

Christopherson, J. (1983) Public perception of child abuse and the need for prevention: are professionals seen as abusers?, *Child Abuse and Neglect*, 7: 435–42.

Cicchetti, D. and Aber, L. (1980) Abused children – abusive parents: an overstated case, *Harvard Educational Review*, 50: 244–55.

Cicchetti, D. and Carlson, V. (eds) (1989) *Child Maltreatment: Theory and Research on the Causes and Consequences of Child Abuse and Neglect*. Cambridge: Cambridge University Press.

Cleaver, H. and Freeman, P. (1995) *Parental Perspectives in Cases of Suspected Child Abuse*. London: HMSO.

Clyde, Lord (1992) *Report of the Inquiry into the Removal of Children from Orkney in February 1991*, HoC 195. London: HMSO.

Cobley, C. (1995) *Child Abuse and the Law*. London: Cavendish.

Cohen, C. and Adler, A. (1986) Assessing the role of social network interventions with an inner-city population, *American Journal of Orthopsychiatry*, 56: 278–88.

Cohen, F. and Densen-Gerber, J. (1982) A study of the relationship between child abuse and drug addiction in 178 parents: preliminary results, *Child Abuse and Neglect*, 6: 383–7.

Cohn, A. and Daro, D. (1987) Is treatment too late? What ten years of evaluative research tell us, *Child Abuse and Neglect*, 11: 433–42.

Collins, S. (ed.) (1990) *Alcohol, Social Work and Helping*. London: Routledge.

Colton, M. and Vanstone, M. (1996) *Betrayal of Trust: Sexual Abuse by Men who Work with Children . . . in their Own Words*. London: Free Association.

Conte, J. and Schuerman, J. (1987) Factors associated with an increased impact of child sexual abuse, *Child Abuse and Neglect*, 11: 201–11.

Coohey, C. (1996) Child maltreatment: testing the social isolation hypothesis, *Child Abuse and Neglect*, 20: 241–54.

Coohey, C. and Braun, N. (1997) Toward an integrated framework for understanding child physical abuse, *Child Abuse and Neglect*, 21: 1081–94.

Cooper, A., Hetherington, R., Baistow, K., Pitts, J. and Spriggs, A. (1995) *Positive Child Protection: A View from Abroad*. Lyme Regis: Russell House.

Corby, B. (1987) *Working with Child Abuse*. Milton Keynes: Open University Press.

Corby, B. (1990) Making use of child protection statistics, *Children and Society*, 4: 304–14.

Corby, B. (1991) Sociology, social work and child protection, in M. Davies (ed.) *The Sociology of Social Work*. London: Routledge.

Corby, B. (1996) Risk assessment in child protection work, in H. Kemshall and J. Pritchard (eds) *Good Practice in Risk Assessment and Risk Management*. London: Jessica Kingsley.

Corby, B. (1998) *Managing Child Sexual Abuse Cases*. London: Jessica Kingsley.

Corby, B. and Cox, P. (1998) The 'new witch-hunters'?, *NOTA News*, 26: 30–2.

Corby, B. and Millar, M. (1997) A parents' view of partnership, in J. Bates, R. Pugh and N. Thompson (eds) *Protecting Children: Challenges and Change*. Aldershot: Avebury Press.

Corby, B. and Mills, C. (1986) Child abuse: risks and resources, *British Journal of Social Work*, 16: 531–42.

Corby, B., Millar, M. and Young, L. (1996) Parental participation in child protection work: rethinking the rhetoric, *British Journal of Social Work*, 26: 475–92.

Corby, B., Doig, A. and Roberts, V. (1998) Inquiries into child abuse, *Journal of Social Welfare and Family Law*, 20: 377–95.

Creighton, S. (1984) *Trends in Child Abuse.* London: NSPCC.

Creighton, S. (1985, 1986, 1987) *Initial Findings from NSPCC Register Research 1984, 1985, 1986.* London: NSPCC.

Creighton, S. (1993) Children's homicide: an exchange, *British Journal of Social Work*, 23: 643–4.

Creighton, S. and Noyes, P. (1989) *Child Abuse Trends in England and Wales 1983–1987.* London: NSPCC.

Crittenden, P. (1983) The effect of mandatory protective day care on mutual attachment in maltreating mother–infant dyads, *Child Abuse and Neglect*, 7: 297–300.

Crittenden, P. and Ainsworth, M. (1989) Child maltreatment and attachment theory, in D. Cicchetti and V. Carlson (eds) *Child Maltreatment: Theory and Research into the Causes and Consequences of Child Abuse and Neglect.* Cambridge: Cambridge University Press.

Crozier, J. and Katz, R. (1979) Social learning treatment of child abuse, *Journal of Behavioral Therapy and Experimental Psychiatry*, 10: 213–20.

Culp, R., Heide, J. and Taylor-Richardson, M. (1987) Maltreated children and developmental scores: treatment versus non-treatment, *Child Abuse and Neglect*, 11: 29–34.

Cunningham, H. (1991) *Children of the Poor.* Oxford: Blackwell.

Curtis, Dame M. (1946) *Report of the Care of Children Committee.* London: HMSO.

Curtis, P. and McCullough, C. (1993) The impact of alcohol and other drugs on the child welfare system, *Child Welfare*, 72: 533–42.

Dale, P., Morrison, T., Davies, M., Noyes, P. and Roberts, W. (1983) A family therapy approach to child abuse: countering resistance, *Journal of Family Therapy*, 5: 117–43.

Dale, P., Davies, M., Morrison, T. and Waters, J. (1986) *Dangerous Families: Assessment and Treatment of Child Abuse.* London: Tavistock.

Davin, A. (1990) The precocity of poverty, in *The Proceedings of the Conference on Historical Perspectives on Childhood.* University of Trondheim.

Dawkins, R. (1976) *The Selfish Gene.* Oxford: Oxford University Press.

Deblinger, E., McLeer, S., Atkins, M., Ralphe, M. and Foa, E. (1989) Post-traumatic stress in sexually abused, physically abused and non-abused children, *Child Abuse and Neglect*, 13: 403–8.

De Francis, V. (1969) *Protecting the Child Victim of Sex Crimes Committed by Adults.* Denver, CO: American Humane Association.

De Mause, L. (ed.) (1976) *The History of Childhood.* London: Souvenir Press.

Demos, J. (1986) *Past, Present and Personal.* Oxford: Oxford University Press.

Denicola, J. and Sandler, J. (1980) Training abusive parents in child management and self-control skills, *Behavior Therapy*, 11: 263–70.

Department of Health (1988) *Protecting Children: A Guide for Social Workers Undertaking a Comprehensive Assessment.* London: HMSO.

Department of Health (1989, 1990, 1991c, 1992, 1993, 1996, 1999c) *Survey of Children and Young Persons on Child Protection Registers, Year Ending 31 March 1988, 1989, 1990, 1991, 1992, 1995, 1999 England.* London: HMSO.

Department of Health (1991a) *Child Abuse: A Study of Inquiry Reports 1980–1989.* London: HMSO.

Department of Health (1991b) *Working Together under the Children Act 1989: A Guide to Arrangements for Inter-agency Cooperation for the Protection of Children from Abuse.* London: HMSO.

Department of Health (1995) *Child Protection: Messages from Research*. London: HMSO.

Department of Health (1998a) *Caring for Children away from Home: Messages from Research*. Chichester: Wiley.

Department of Health (1998b) *The Quality Protects Programme: Transforming Children's Services*, LAC(98)26. London: Department of Health.

Department of Health (1998c) *Modernising Social Services: Promoting Independence, Improving Protection, Raising Standards*. London: The Stationery Office.

Department of Health (2000a) *Working Together to Safeguard Children: A Guide to Inter-agency Working to Safeguard and Promote the Welfare of Children*. London: The Stationery Office.

Department of Health (2000b) *Framework for the Assessment of Children in Need and their Families*. London: The Stationery Office.

Department of Health and Social Security (1974) *Report of the Committee of Inquiry into the Care and Supervision Provided in Relation to Maria Colwell*. London: HMSO.

Department of Health and Social Security (1975) *Report of the Committee of Inquiry into the Provision of Services to the Family of John George Auckland*. London: HMSO.

Department of Health and Social Security (1978) *Report of the Social Work Service of the DHSS into Certain Aspects of the Management of the Case of Stephen Menheniott*. London: HMSO.

Department of Health and Social Security (1979) *The Report of the Committee of Inquiry into the Actions of the Authorities and Agencies Relating to Darryn James Clarke*, Cmnd 7739. London: HMSO.

Department of Health and Social Security (1980) *Child Abuse: Central Register Systems*, LASSL (80)4. London: HMSO.

Department of Health and Social Security (1982) *Child Abuse: A Study of Inquiry Reports 1973–1981*. London: HMSO.

Department of Health and Social Security (1985a) *Social Work Decisions in Child Care: Recent Research Findings and their Implications*. London: HMSO.

Department of Health and Social Security (1985b) *Review of Child Care Law: Report to Ministers of an Interdepartmental Working Party*. London: HMSO.

Department of Health and Social Security (1986) *Child Abuse – Working Together: A Draft Guide to Arrangements for Inter-agency Cooperation for the Protection of Children*. London: HMSO.

Department of Health and Social Security (1988) *Working Together: A Guide to Inter-agency Cooperation for the Protection of Children from Abuse*. London: HMSO.

Department of Health and Social Security (Northern Ireland) (1985) *Report of the Committee of Inquiry into Children's Homes and Hostels*. Belfast: HMSO.

Dibble, J. and Straus, M. (1980) Some structural determinants of inconsistency between attitudes and behavior: the case of family violence, *Journal of Marriage and the Family*, 42: 71–82.

Dickens, J. (1993) Assessment and control of social work: an analysis of the reasons for the non-use of the child assessment order, *Journal of Social Welfare and Family Law*, 15: 88–100.

Dingwall, R. (1989) Some problems about predicting child abuse and neglect, in O. Stevenson (ed.) *Child Abuse: Public Policy and Professional Practice*. Hemel Hempstead: Harvester-Wheatsheaf.

Dingwall, R., Eekelaar, J. and Murray, T. (1983) *The Protection of Children: State Intervention and Family Life*. Oxford: Blackwell.

Dingwall, R., Eekelaar, J. and Murray, T. (1984) Childhood as a social problem: a survey of the history of legal regulation, *Journal of Law and Society*, 11: 207–32.

Dobash, R. and Dobash, R. (1992) *Women, Violence and Social Change*. London: Routledge.

Dominelli, L. (1986) Father–daughter incest: patriarchy's shameful secret, *Critical Social Policy*, 16: 8–22.

Donnison, D. (1954) *The Neglected Child and the Social Services*. Manchester: Manchester University Press.

Donzelot, J. (1980) *The Policing of Families: Welfare versus the State*. London: Hutchinson.

Dore, M., Doris, J. and Wright, P. (1995) Identifying substance abuse in maltreating families: a child welfare challenge, *Child Abuse and Neglect*, 19: 531–43.

Driver, E. and Droisen, A. (eds) (1989) *Child Sexual Abuse: Feminist Perspectives*. London: Macmillan.

Dubanoski, R., Evans, I. and Higuchi, A. (1978) Analysis and treatment of child abuse: a set of behavioral propositions, *Child Abuse and Neglect*, 2: 153–72.

Egeland, B. (1988) Breaking the cycle of abuse: implications for prediction and intervention, in K. Browne, C. Davies and P. Stratton (eds) *Early Prediction and Prevention of Child Abuse*. Chichester: Wiley.

Egeland, B. and Vaughan, B. (1981) Failure of bond formation as a cause of abuse, neglect and maltreatment, *American Journal of Orthopsychiatry*, 51: 78–84.

Egeland, B., Sroufe, L. and Erickson, M. (1983) Developmental consequences of different patterns of maltreatment, *Child Abuse and Neglect*, 7: 459–69.

Elbedour, S., ten Bensel, R. and Bastien, D. (1993) Ecological integrated model of children at war: individual and social psychology, *Child Abuse and Neglect*, 17: 805–19.

Elders, J. (1999) The call to action, *Child Abuse and Neglect*, 23: 1003–9.

Elliott, M., Browne, K. and Kilcoyne, J. (1995) Child sexual abuse prevention: what offenders tell us, *Child Abuse and Neglect*, 19: 579–94.

Elmer, E. (1977) *Fragile Families, Troubled Children*. Pittsburgh, PA: University of Pittsburgh Press.

Elwell, M. and Ephloss, P. (1987) Initial reactions of sexually abused children, *Social Casework*, 68: 109–16.

Ennew, J. (1986) *The Sexual Exploitation of Children*. Cambridge: Polity Press.

Erickson, M., Egeland, B. and Pianta, R. (1989) Effects of maltreatment on the development of young children, in D. Cicchetti and V. Carlson (eds) *Child Maltreatment: Theory and Research on the Causes and Consequences of Child Abuse and Neglect*. Cambridge: Cambridge University Press.

Erooga, M. and Masson, H. (1999) *Children and Young People Who Sexually Abuse Others: Challenges and Responses*. London: Routledge.

Everson, M. and Boat, B. (1994) Putting the anatomical doll controversy in perspective: an examination of the major uses and criticisms of the dolls in child sexual abuse evaluations, *Child Abuse and Neglect*, 18: 113–29.

Falkov, A. (1996) *Study of Working Together 'Part 8' Reports: Fatal Child Abuse and Parental Psychiatric Disorder: An Analysis of 100 Area Child Protection Committee Case Reviews under the Children Act 1989*. London: Department of Health.

Faller, K. (1989) Why sexual abuse? An exploration of the intergenerational hypothesis, *Child Abuse and Neglect*, 13: 543–8.

Fancher, R. (1973) *Psychoanalytic Psychology: The Development of Freud's Thought*. London: Norton.

Farmer, E. (1992) Restoring children on court orders to their families: lessons for practice, *Adoption and Fostering*, 16: 7–15.

Farmer, E. and Owen, M. (1995) *Child Protection Practice: Private Risks and Public Remedies: a Study of Decision-making, Intervention and Outcome in Child Protection Work*. London: HMSO.

Featherstone, B. and Lancaster, E. (1997) Contemplating the unthinkable: men who sexually abuse children, *Critical Social Policy*, 17: 51–68.

Fehrenbach, P. and Monastersky, C. (1988) Characteristics of female adolescent sexual offenders, *American Journal of Orthopsychiatry*, 58: 148–51.

Fehrenbach, P., Smith, W., Monastersky, C. and Deister, R. (1986) Adolescent sex offenders: offender and offense characteristics, *American Journal of Orthopsychiatry*, 56: 225–33.

Ferguson, D. and Lynsky, M. (1996) Physical punishment/maltreatment during childhood and adjustment in young adulthood, *Child Abuse and Neglect*, 20: 617–30.

Ferguson, H. (1990) Rethinking child protection practices: a case for history, in The Violence against Children Study Group, *Taking Child Abuse Seriously*. London: Unwin Hyman.

Fielding, N. and Conroy, S. (1992) Interviewing child victims: police and social work investigations of child sexual abuse, *Sociology*, 26: 103–24.

Finkelhor, D. (1979) *Sexually Victimized Children*. New York: Free Press.

Finkelhor, D. (1984) *Child Sexual Abuse: New Theory and Research*. New York: Free Press.

Finkelhor, D. (1993) Epidemiological factors in the clinical identification of child sexual abuse, *Child Abuse and Neglect*, 17: 67–70.

Finkelhor, D. (1994) The international epidemiology of child sexual abuse, *Child Abuse and Neglect*, 18: 409–17.

Finkelhor, D. and Baron, L. (1986) High risk children, in D. Finkelhor *et al.* (eds) *A Sourcebook on Child Sexual Abuse*. Newbury Park, CA: Sage.

Finkelhor, D. and Korbin, J. (1988) Child abuse as an international issue, *Child Abuse and Neglect*, 12: 3–23.

Finkelhor, D. with Araji, S. *et al.* (eds) (1986) *A Sourcebook on Child Sexual Abuse*. Newbury Park, CA: Sage.

Finkelhor, D., Hotaling, G., Lewis, I. and Smith, C. (1990) Sexual abuse in a national survey of adult men and women: prevalence characteristics and risk factors, *Child Abuse and Neglect*, 14: 19–28.

Finkelhor, D., Asdigan, N. and Dziuba-Leatherman, J. (1995) The effectiveness of victimization prevention instruction: an evaluation of children's responses to actual threats and assaults, *Child Abuse and Neglect*, 19: 141–53.

Fischer, D. and Macdonald, W. (1998) Characteristics of intrafamilial and extrafamilial child sexual abuse, *Child Abuse and Neglect*, 22: 915–29.

Flin, R. (1990) Child witnesses in criminal courts, *Children and Society*, 4: 264–83.

Fox-Harding, L. (1991) *Perspectives in Child Care Policy*. London: Longman.

Fox-Harding, L. (1996) *Family, State and Social Policy*. London: Macmillan.

Freeman, M. (1983) *The Rights and Wrongs of Children*. London: Pinter.

Freeman, M. (1988) Time to stop hitting our children, *Childright*, 51: 5–8.

Freeman, M. (1999) Children are unbeatable, *Children and Society*, 13: 130–41.

Frenken, J. (1994) Treatment of incest perpetrators; a five-phase model, *Child Abuse and Neglect*, 18: 357–65.

Friedrich, J. and Boriskin, J. (1976) The role of the child in abuse: a review of the literature, *American Journal of Orthopsychiatry*, 46: 580–9.

Friedrich, W. (1979) Predictors of coping behaviour of mothers of handicapped children, *Journal of Consulting and Clinical Psychology*, 47: 1140–1.

Friedrich, W., Urquiza, A. and Beilke, R. (1986) Behaviour problems in sexually abused young children, *Journal of Pediatric Psychology*, 11: 47–57.

Frodi, A. and Lamb, M. (1980) Child abusers' response to infant smiles and cries, *Child Development*, 51: 238–41.

Frodi, A. and Smetana, J. (1984) Abused, neglected and non-maltreated preschoolers' ability to discriminate emotion in others: the effects of IQ, *Child Abuse and Neglect*, 8: 459–65.

Fromuth, M. (1986) The relationship of childhood sexual abuse with later psychological and sexual adjustment in a sample of college women, *Child Abuse and Neglect*, 10: 5–15.

Frost, N. and Stein, M. (1989) *The Politics of Child Welfare: Inequality, Power and Change*. Hemel Hempstead: Harvester-Wheatsheaf.

Furby, L., Weinrott, W. and Blackshaw, L. (1989) Sex offender recidivism: a review, *Psychological Bulletin*, 105: 3–30.

Furniss, T. (1991) *The Multi-professional Handbook of Child Sexual Abuse: Integrated Management, Therapy and Legal Intervention*. London: Routledge.

Gabinet, L. (1983a) Child abuse treatment failures reveal need for redefinition of the problem, *Child Abuse and Neglect*, 7: 395–402.

Gabinet, L. (1983b) Shared parenting: a new paradigm for the treatment of child abuse, *Child Abuse and Neglect*, 7: 403–11.

Gagnon, J. and Parker, R. (1995) *Conceiving Sexuality: Approaches to Sex Research in the Modern World*. London: Routledge.

Garbarino, J. (1977) The human ecology of child maltreatment: a conceptual model for research, *Journal of Marriage and the Family*, 39: 721–35.

Garbarino, J. (1982) *Children and Families in their Social Environment*. New York: Aldine.

Garbarino, J. and Crouter, A. (1978) Defining the community context for parent–child relations: the correlates of child mistreatment, *Child Development*, 49: 604–16.

Garbarino, J. and Gilliam, G. (1980) *Understanding Abusive Families*. Lexington, MA: Lexington Books.

Garbarino, J. and Vondra, J. (1987) Psychological maltreatment: issues and perspectives, in M. Brassard, R. Germain and S. Hart (eds) *Psychological Maltreatment of Children and Youth*. Oxford: Pergamon Press.

Gardner, L. (1972) Deprivation dwarfism, *Scientific American*, 227: 76–82.

Gelles, R. (1982) Towards better research on child abuse and neglect: a response to Besharov, *Child Abuse and Neglect*, 6: 495–6.

Gelles, R. (1989) Child abuse and violence in single parent families: parent absence and economic deprivation, *American Journal of Orthopsychiatry*, 59: 492–501.

Gelles, R. and Cornell, C. (1985) *Intimate Violence in Families*. Beverly Hills, CA: Sage.

Gelles, R. and Edfeldt, A. (1986) Violence towards children in the United States and Sweden, *Child Abuse and Neglect*, 10: 501–10.

George, C. and Main, M. (1979) Social interaction of young abused children: approach, avoidance and aggression, *Child Development*, 50: 306–18.

Germain, C. and Gitterman, A. (1980) *The Life Model of Social Work Practice*. Cambridge, MA: Harvard University Press.

Giaretto, H. (1981) A comprehensive child sexual abuse treatment program, in P. Mrazek and C. Kempe (eds) *Sexually Abused Children and their Families*. New York: Pergamon Press.

Giaretto, H., Giaretto, A. and Sgroi, S. (1978) Co-ordinated community treatment of incest, in A. Burgess, A. Groth, L. Holmstrom and S. Sgroi (eds) *Sexual Assault of Children and Adolescents*. Lexington, MA: Lexington Books.

Gibbons, J., Conroy, S. and Bell, C. (1995a) *Operating the Child Protection System: A Study of Child Protection Practices in English Local Authorities*. London: HMSO.

Gibbons, J., Gallagher, B., Bell, C. and Gordon, D. (1995b) *Development after Physical Abuse in Early Childhood: A Follow-Up Study of Children on Child Protection Registers*. London: HMSO.

Gil, D. (1970) *Violence Against Children*. Cambridge, MA: Harvard University Press.

Gil, D. (1975) Unravelling child abuse, *American Journal of Orthopsychiatry*, 45: 346–56.

Gil, D. (1978) Societal violence and violence in families, in J. Eekelaar and S. Katz (eds) *Family Violence*. Toronto: Butterworth.

Gillham, B. (1991) *The Facts about Sexual Abuse*. London: Cassell.

Giovannoni, J. and Becerra, R. (1979) *Defining Child Abuse*. New York: Free Press.

Giovannoni, J. and Billingsley, A. (1970) Child neglect among the poor: a study of parental adequacy in families of three ethnic groups, *Child Welfare*, 49: 196–204.

Glaser, D. and Frosh, S. (1988) *Child Sexual Abuse*. London: Macmillan.

Gold, S., Hughes, D. and Swingle, J. (1996) Characteristics of childhood sexual abuse among female survivors in therapy, *Child Abuse and Neglect*, 20: 323–36.

Goldstein, J., Freud, A. and Solnit, A. (1979) *Beyond the Best Interests of the Child*. New York: Free Press.

Goldston, D., Turnquist, D. and Knutson, J. (1989) Presenting problems of sexually abused girls receiving psychiatric services, *Journal of Abnormal Psychology*, 98: 547–60.

Gomes-Schwartz, B., Horowitz, J. and Cardarelli, A. (1990) *Child Sexual Abuse: The Initial Effects*. Beverly Hills, CA: Sage.

Goode, W. (1971) Force and violence in the family, *Journal of Marriage and the Family*, 33: 624–36.

Goodwin, J., McCarthy, T. and DiVasto, P. (1981) Prior incest in mothers of abused children, *Child Abuse and Neglect*, 7: 163–70.

Gordon, L. (1989) *Heroes of their Own Lives: The Politics and History of Family Violence, Boston 1880–1960*. London: Virago.

Gordon, M. and Creighton, S. (1988) Natal and non-natal fathers as sexual abusers in the UK: a comparative analysis, *Journal of Marriage and the Family*, 50: 99–105.

Gorham, D. (1978) The maiden tribute of Babylon reexamined: child prostitution and the idea of childhood in late-Victorian England, *Victorian Studies*, 21: 354–79.

Gough, D. (1988) Approaches to child abuse prevention, in K. Browne, J. Davies and P. Stratton (eds) *Early Prediction and Prevention of Child Abuse.* Chichester: Wiley.

Gough, D. (1993) *Child Abuse Interventions: A Review of the Research Literature.* London: HMSO.

Gough, D. (1996) Defining the problem, *Child Abuse and Neglect*, 20: 993–1002.

Gray, J. and Ben-Tovim, A. (1996) Illness induction syndrome: paper 1 – a series of 41 children from 37 families identified at the Great Ormond Street Hospital for Children, NHS Trust, *Child Abuse and Neglect*, 20: 654–72.

Gray, J., Cutler, C., Dean, J. and Kempe, C. (1977) Prediction and prevention of child abuse and neglect, *Child Abuse and Neglect*, 1: 45–58.

Green, A., Power, E., Steinbok, B. and Gaines, R. (1981) Factors associated with successful and unsuccessful intervention with child abusive families, *Child Abuse and Neglect*, 5: 45–52.

Greenland, C. (1958) Incest, *British Journal of Delinquency*, 9: 62–5.

Greenland, C. (1987) *Preventing CAN Deaths: An International Study of Deaths Due to Child Abuse and Neglect.* London: Tavistock.

Greenwalt, B., Sklare, G. and Portes, P. (1998) The therapeutic treatment provided in cases involving physical child abuse: a description of current practices, *Child Abuse and Neglect*, 22: 71–8.

Greenwich (London Borough of) (1987) *A Child in Mind: The Protection of Children in a Responsible Society. Report of the Commission of Inquiry into the Circumstances Surrounding the Death of Kimberley Carlile.* London: London Borough of Greenwich.

Griffiths, D. and Moynihan, F. (1963) Multiple epiphyseal injuries in babies ('battered baby syndrome'), *British Medical Journal*, 5372: 1558–61.

Groth, A. and Burgess, A. (1979) Sexual traumas in the life histories of rapists and child molesters, *Victimology*, 4: 10–16.

Hallett, C. and Stevenson, O. (1980) *Child Abuse: Aspects of Interprofessional Cooperation.* London: Allen & Unwin.

Halston, A. and Richards, D. (1982) Behind closed doors, *Social Work Today*, 14: 7–11.

Hampton, R., Gelles, R. and Harrop, J. (1989) Is violence in black families increasing? A comparison of 1975 and 1985 national survey rates, *Journal of Marriage and the Family*, 89: 969–80.

Hanawalt, B. (1977) Childrearing among the lower classes of late medieval England, *Journal of Interdisciplinary History*, 8: 1–22.

Harris, R. (1995) Child protection, child care and child welfare, in J. Wilson and A. James (eds) *The Child Protection Handbook.* London: Baillière-Tindall.

Harrison, P., Falkerson, J. and Beebe, T. (1996) Multiple substance use among adolescent physical and sexual abuse victims, *Child Abuse and Neglect*, 19: 529–39.

Harrow (Area Child Protection Committee) (1999) *Part 8 Summary Report.* Harrow: Harrow ACPC.

Hearn, J. (1990) Child abuse and men's violence, in The Violence against Children Study Group, *Taking Child Abuse Seriously.* London: Unwin Hyman.

Hendrick, H. (1994) *Child Welfare: England 1872–1989.* London: Routledge.

Henning, K., Leitenberg, H., Coffey, P., Bennett, T. and Jankowski, M. (1997) Long-term psychological adjustment to witnessing interparental physical conflict during childhood, *Child Abuse and Neglect*, 21: 501–15.

Hensey, O., Williams, J. and Rosenbloom, L. (1983) Intervention in child abuse: experience in Liverpool, *Developmental Medicine and Child Neurology*, 25: 606–11.

Herman, J. (1981) *Father–Daughter Incest*. Cambridge, MA: Harvard University Press.

Higginson, S. (1992) Decision-making in the assessment of risk in child abuse cases. Unpublished MPhil thesis, Cranfield Institute of Technology.

Hillingdon (London Borough of) (1986) *Report of the Review Panel into the Death of Heidi Koseda*. London: London Borough of Hillingdon.

Hobbs, C. and Wynne, J. (1986) Buggery in childhood: a common syndrome of child abuse, *The Lancet*, 8510: 792–6.

Hoffman-Plotkin, D. and Twentyman, C. (1984) A multimodal assessment of behavioral and cognitive deficits in abused and neglected pre-schoolers, *Child Development*, 55: 794–802.

Holman, B. (1988) *Putting Families First: Prevention and Child Care*. London: Macmillan.

Holmes, S. (1978) Parents anonymous: a treatment method for child abuse, *Social Work*, 23: 245–7.

Holt, J. (1974) *Escape from Childhood*. Harmondsworth: Penguin.

Home Office (1923) *Report of the Work of the Children's Branch*. London: HMSO.

Home Office (1945) *Report by Sir Walter Monckton on the Circumstances which Led to the Boarding-out of Dennis and Terence O'Neill at Bank Farm, Minsterley and the Steps Taken to Supervise their Welfare*, Cmd 6636. London: HMSO.

Home Office (1950) *Children Neglected or Ill-treated in their Own Homes*. Joint Circular with the Ministry of Health and Ministry of Education. London: HMSO.

Home Office/Department of Health (1992) *Memorandum of Good Practice on Video-Recorded Interviews with Child Witnesses for Criminal Proceedings*. London: HMSO.

Hooper, C-A. (1992) *Mothers Surviving Child Sexual Abuse*. London: Tavistock.

Houlbrooke, R. (1984) *The English Family 1450–1700*. London: Longman.

Housden, L. (1955) *The Prevention of Cruelty to Children*. London: Cape.

House of Commons (1984) *Children in Care Volume 1. Second Report from the Social Services Committee: Session 1983–4*. London: HMSO.

Howe, D. (1980) Inflated states and empty theories in social work, *British Journal of Social Work*, 10: 317–40.

Howe, D. (1991) Knowledge, power and the shape of social work practice, in M. Davies (ed.) *The Sociology of Social Work*. London: Routledge.

Howe, D. (1995) *Attachment Theory for Social Work Practice*. London: Macmillan.

Howe, Lady (1992) *The Quality of Care: Report of the Residential Staff's Inquiry*. London: Local Government Management Board.

Howes, C. and Espinosa, M. (1985) The consequences of child abuse for the formation of relationships with peers, *Child Abuse and Neglect*, 9: 397–404.

Hoyles, M. (1979) Childhood in historical perspective, in M. Hoyles (ed.) *Changing Childhood*. London: Writers and Readers Publishing Cooperative.

Hrdy, S. (1977) *The Langurs of Abu*. Cambridge, MA: Harvard University Press.

Humphreys, C. (1995) Whatever happened on the way to counselling? Hurdles in the interagency environment, *Child Abuse and Neglect*, 19: 801–9.

Hunt, D. (1970) *Parents and Children in History*. New York: Basic Books.

Hunt, P. (1994) *Report of the Independent Inquiry into Multiple Abuse in Nursery Classes in Newcastle-upon-Tyne*. Newcastle upon Tyne: City Council of Newcastle upon Tyne.

Hunter, R. and Kilstrom, N. (1979) Breaking the cycle in abusive families, *American Journal of Psychiatry*, 136: 1320–2.

Hyman, C. (1978) Some characteristics of abusing families referred to the NSPCC, *British Journal of Social Work*, 8: 629–35.

Ingleby, Viscount (1960) *Report of the Committee on Children and Young Persons*, Cmnd 1191. London: HMSO.

Isaacs, C. (1982) Treatment of child abuse: a review of behavioral interventions, *Journal of Applied Behavioral Analysis*, 15: 273–94.

Iwaniec, D. (1997) Evaluating parent training for emotionally abusive and neglectful parents: comparing individual versus individual and group intervention, *Research on Social Work Practice*, 7: 329–49.

Iwaniec, D., Herbert, M. and McNeish, A. (1985) Social work with failure to thrive children and their families: part II: behavioural social work intervention, *British Journal of Social Work*, 15: 375–89.

Jackson, S. (1996) Educational success for looked-after children: the social worker's responsibility, *Practice*, 10: 47–56.

Jacobson, R. and Straker, G. (1982) Peer group interaction of physically abused children, *Child Abuse and Neglect*, 6: 321–7.

Jahoda, M. (1977) *Freud and the Dilemmas of Psychology*. London: Hogarth Press.

Jampole, L. and Weber, M. (1987) An assessment of the behaviour of sexually abused and nonsexually abused children with anatomically correct dolls, *Child Abuse and Neglect*, 11: 187–92.

Jaudes, P. and Diamond, L. (1985) The handicapped child and child abuse, *Child Abuse and Neglect*, 9: 341–7.

Jaudes, P. and Morris, M. (1990) Child sexual abuse: who goes home?, *Child Abuse and Neglect*, 14: 61–8.

Jayaratne, S. (1977) Child abusers as parents and children: a review, *Social Work*, 22: 5–9.

Jenkins, H. and Asen, K. (1992) Family therapy without the family: a framework for systemic practice, *Journal of Family Therapy*, 14: 1–14.

Jesson, J. (1993) Understanding adolescent female prostitution: a literature review, *British Journal of Social Work*, 23: 517–30.

Johnson, T. (1988) Child perpetrators: children who molest other children: preliminary findings, *Child Abuse and Neglect*, 12: 219–29.

Johnson, T. (1989) Female child perpetrators: children who molest other children, *Child Abuse and Neglect*, 13: 571–86.

Johnston, M. (1979) The sexually mistreated child: diagnostic evaluation, *Child Abuse and Neglect*, 3: 943–51.

Jones, D. (1987) The untreatable family, *Child Abuse and Neglect*, 11: 409–20.

Jordanova, L. (1989) Children in history: concepts of nature and society, in G. Scarre (ed.) *Children, Parents and Politics*. Cambridge: Cambridge University Press.

Joseph, Sir Keith (1972) The next ten years, *New Society*, 5 October: 8–9.

Kadushin, A. and Martin, J. (1981) *Child Abuse: An Interactional Event*. New York: Columbia University Press.

Kaufman, J. and Zigler, E. (1987) Do abused children become abusive parents?, *American Journal of Orthopsychiatry*, 57: 186–92.

Kaufman, J. and Zigler, E. (1989) The intergenerational transmission of child abuse, in D. Cicchetti and V. Carlson (eds) *Child Maltreatment: Theory and Research on the Causes and Consequences of Child Abuse and Neglect*. Cambridge: Cambridge University Press.

Kelly, L. (1988) *Surviving Sexual Violence*. Cambridge: Polity Press.

Kelly, L., Regan, L. and Burton, S. (1991) *An Exploratory Study of the Prevalence of Sexual Abuse in a Sample of 16–21 Year Olds*. London: Child Abuse Studies Unit, University of North London.

Kempe, C., Silverman, F., Steele, B., Droegemueller, W. and Silver, H. (1962) The battered child syndrome, *Journal of the American Medical Association*, 181: 17–24.

Kempe, R. and Kempe, C. (1978) *Child Abuse*. London: Fontana.

Kendall-Tackett, K. and Eckenrode, J. (1996) The effects of neglect on academic achievement and disciplinary problems: a developmental perspective, *Child Abuse and Neglect*, 20: 161–9.

Kilgallon, W. (1995) *Report of the Independent Review into Allegations of Abuse at Meadowdale Children's Home and Related Matters*. Morpeth: Northumberland County Council.

Kinard, E. (1980) Mental health needs of abused children, *Child Welfare*, 49: 45–62.

King, J. and Taitz, L. (1985) Catch-up growth following abuse, *Archives of Disease in Childhood*, 60: 1152–4.

Kline, P. (1981) *Fact and Fantasy in Freudian Theory*. London: Methuen.

Kolko, J., Moser, J. and Weldy, S. (1988) Behavioral/emotional indicators of sexual abuse in child psychiatric in-patients: a controlled comparison with physical abuse, *Child Abuse and Neglect*, 12: 529–41.

Korbin, J. (ed.) (1981) *Child Abuse and Neglect: Cross Cultural Perspectives*. Berkeley, CA: University of California Press.

Korbin, J. (1989) Fatal maltreatment by mothers: a proposed framework, *Child Abuse and Neglect*, 13: 481–9.

Koreola, C., Pound, J., Heger, A. and Lyttle, C. (1993) Relationship of child sexual abuse to depression, *Child Abuse and Neglect*, 17: 393–400.

Krug, R. (1989) Adult male report of childhood sexual abuse by mothers: case descriptions, motivations and long-term consequences, *Child Abuse and Neglect*, 13: 111–19.

Krugman, R. (1991) Child abuse and neglect: critical first steps in response to a national emergency, *American Journal of Diseases in Childhood*, 145: 513–15.

Krugman, R. (1998) Keynote address: it's time to broaden the agenda, *Child Abuse and Neglect*, 22: 475–9.

Kumar, V. (1993) *Poverty and Inequality in the UK: The Effects on Children*. London: National Children's Bureau.

La Fontaine, J. (1988) *Child Sexual Abuse: An ESRC Research Briefing*. London: Economic and Social Research Council.

La Fontaine, J. (1990) *Child Sexual Abuse*. Cambridge: Polity Press.

La Fontaine, J. (1994) *The Extent and Nature of Organised and Ritual Abuse: Research Findings*. London: HMSO.

La Fontaine, J. (1998) *Speak of the Devil: Tales of Satanic Abuse in Contemporary England*. Cambridge: Cambridge University Press.

Lambeth (London Borough of) (1987) *Whose Child? The Report of the Public Inquiry into the Death of Tyra Henry*. London: London Borough of Lambeth.

Lambeth, Lewisham and Southwark (London Boroughs of) (1989) *The Doreen Aston Report*. London: Lambeth, Lewisham and Southwark Area Review Committee.

Lamphear, V. (1985) The impact of maltreatment on children's psychosocial adjustment: a review of the research, *Child Abuse and Neglect*, 9: 251–63.

Larrance, D. and Twentyman, C. (1983) Maternal attribution and child abuse, *Journal of Abnormal Psychology*, 92: 449–57.

Lauderdale, M., Valrunas, A. and Anderson, M. (1980) Race, ethnicity and child maltreatment: an empirical analysis, *Child Abuse and Neglect*, 4: 163–9.

Lawson, C. (1993) Mother–son sexual abuse: rare or underreported? A critique of the research, *Child Abuse and Neglect*, 17: 261–9.

Leach, P. (1999) *The Physical Punishment of Children: Some Input from Recent Research*. London: NSPCC.

Lealman, C., Haigh, D., Phillips, J., Stone, J. and Ord-Smith, C. (1983) Prediction and prevention of child abuse – an empty hope?, *The Lancet*, 8339: 1423–4.

Leicestershire (County Council) (1993) *The Leicestershire Inquiry*. Leicester: Leicestershire County Council.

Letourneau, C. (1981) Empathy and stress: how they affect parental aggression, *Social Work*, 26: 383–90.

Leventhal, J. (1996) Twenty years later: we do know how to prevent child abuse and neglect, *Child Abuse and Neglect*, 20: 647–53.

Leventhal, J., Egester, E. and Murphy, J. (1984) Reassessment of the relationship of perinatal risk factors and child abuse, *American Journal of Diseases in Childhood*, 138: 1034–9.

Lewis, D., Mallouh, C. and Webb, V. (1989) Child abuse, delinquency and violent criminality, in D. Cicchetti and V. Carlson (eds) *Child Maltreatment: Theory and Research on the Causes and Consequences of Child Abuse and Neglect*. Cambridge: Cambridge University Press.

Lewis, M. and Schaeffer, S. (1981) Peer behaviour and mother–infant interaction, in M. Lewis and S. Schaeffer (eds) *The Uncommon Child*. New York: Plenum Press.

Lewisham (London Borough of) (1985) *The Leeways Inquiry Report*. London: London Borough of Lewisham.

Lindberg, F. and Distad, L. (1985) Survival reponses to incest: adolescents in crisis, *Child Abuse and Neglect*, 9: 413–15.

Lindon, J. and Nourse, C. (1994) A multi-dimensional model of groupwork for adolescent girls who have been sexually abused, *Child Abuse and Neglect*, 18: 341–8.

Lindsey, D. and Trocme, N. (1994) Have child protection efforts reduced child homicides? An examination of the data from Britain and North America, *British Journal of Social Work*, 24: 715–32.

Lowe, N. (1989) The role of wardship in child care cases, *Family Law*, 19: 38–45.

Lukianowicz, N. (1971) Battered children, *Psychiatrica Clinica*, 4: 257–80.

Lusk, R. and Waterman, J. (1986) Effects of sexual abuse on children, in K. Macfarlane and J. Waterman (eds) *The Sexual Abuse of Young Children*. New York: Holt, Rinehart & Winston.

Lynch, M. (1975) Ill health and child abuse, *The Lancet*, 7929: 317–19.

Lynch, M. (1988) The consequences of child abuse, in K. Browne, C. Davies and P. Stratton (eds) *Early Prediction and Prevention of Child Abuse*. Chichester: Wiley.

Lynch, M. and Roberts, J. (1977) Predicting child abuse: signs of bonding failure in the maternity hospital, *British Medical Journal*, 6061: 624–6.

Lynch, M. and Roberts, J. (1978) Early alerting signs, in A. Franklin (ed.) *Child Abuse: Prediction, Prevention and Follow-up*. Edinburgh: Churchill Livingstone.

Lynch, M. and Roberts, J. (1982) *The Consequences of Child Abuse*. London: Academic Press.

Lyon, C. (1989) Legal developments following the Cleveland report in England: a consideration of some aspects of the Children Bill, *Journal of Social Welfare Law*, 11: 200–6.

Lyon, C. (1997) Children abused within the care system: do current representation procedures offer the child protection and the family support?, in N. Parton (ed.) *Child Protection and Family Support: Tensions, Contradictions and Possibilities*. London: Routledge.

McAuley, R. and McAuley, P. (1977) *Child Behaviour Problems: An Empirical Guide to Management*. London: Macmillan.

McClure, R. (1981) *Coram's Children: The London Foundling Hospital in the Eighteenth Century*. New Haven, CT: Yale University Press.

McCord, J. (1983) A 40 year perspective on the effects of child abuse and neglect, *Child Abuse and Neglect*, 7: 265–70.

Macdonald, I. (1990) *Murder in the Playground: The Burnage Report*. London: Longsight Press.

Macdonald, K. (1995) Comparative homicide and the proper aims of social work: a sceptical note, *British Journal of Social Work*, 25: 489–97.

Macfarlane, A. (1970) *The Family Life of Ralph Josselin*. Cambridge: Cambridge University Press.

Macfarlane, A. (1979) 'The family, sex and marriage in England 1500–1800' by Laurence Stone, *History and Theory*, 18: 103–26.

Macfarlane, K. and Waterman, J. (1986) *The Sexual Abuse of Young Children*. New York: Holt, Rinehart and Winston.

Mackenzie, T., Collins, N. and Popkin, M. (1982) A case of fetal abuse?, *American Journal of Orthopsychiatry*, 52: 699–703.

Macleod, M. and Saraga, E. (1988) Challenging the orthodoxy: towards a feminist theory and practice, *Feminist Review*, 28: 15–55.

Macpherson, Sir W. (1999) *The Stephen Lawrence Inquiry*. London: The Stationery Office.

Maestripieri, D., Wallen, K. and Carroll, K. (1997) Infant abuse runs in families of group-living Pigtail Macaques, *Child Abuse and Neglect*, 21: 465–71.

Main, N. and Goldwyn, R. (1984) Predicting rejection of her infant from mother's representation of her own experience: implications for the abused–abusing intergenerational cycle, *Child Abuse and Neglect*, 8: 203–17.

Maisch, H. (1973) *Incest*. London: André Deutsch.

Mantell, D. (1988) Clarifying erroneous child sexual abuse allegations, *American Journal of Orthopsychiatry*, 58: 618–21.

Marchant, R. and Page, M. (1992) *Bridging the Gap: Child Protection Work and Children with Multiple Disabilities*. London: NSPCC.

Marneffe, C. (1996) Child abuse treatment: a fallow land, *Child Abuse and Neglect*, 20: 379–84.

Marsh, P. and Crowe, G. (1998) *Family Group Conferences in Child Welfare*. Oxford: Blackwell.

Martin, H. (1972) The child and his development, in C. Kempe and R. Helfer (eds) *Helping the Battered Child and his Family*. Philadelphia, PA: Lippincott.

Martin, J. (1978) Family violence and social policy, in J. Martin (ed.) *Violence and the Family*. Chichester: Wiley.

Martin, J. and Elmer, E. (1992) Battered children grown up: a follow-up study of individuals severely maltreated as children, *Child Abuse and Neglect*, 16: 75–87.

Masson, H. and Erooga, M. (1999) Children and young people who sexually abuse others: incidence, characteristics, causation, in M. Erooga and H. Masson (eds) *Children and Young People who Sexually Abuse Others: Challenges and Responses*. London: Routledge.

Masson, H. and O'Byrne, P. (1990) The family system approach: a help or hindrance?, in The Violence against Children Study Group, *Taking Child Abuse Seriously*. London: Unwin Hyman.

Masson, Jeffrey (1984) *Freud: The Assault on Truth*. London: Faber and Faber.

Masson, Judith (1997) Introducing non-punitive approaches into child protection, in N. Parton (ed.) *Child Protection and Family Support: Tensions, Contradictions and Possibilities*. London: Routledge.

Mayhew, P., Manning, A. and Mirrlees-Black, C. (1993) *The 1992 British Crime Survey: A Home Office Research Unit and Planning Unit Report*. London: HMSO.

Meadow, R. (1977) Munchausen syndrome by proxy: the hinterland of child abuse, *The Lancet*, 57: 92–8.

Meadow, R. (1985) Management of Munchausen syndrome by proxy, *Archives of Disease in Childhood*, 60: 385–93.

Meadow, R. (1989) Suffocation, *British Medical Journal*, 298: 1572–3.

Medden, B. (1985) The assessment of risk: child abuse and neglect case investigations, *Child Abuse and Neglect*, 9: 57–62.

Mehl, A., Coble, L. and Johnson, S. (1990) Munchausen syndrome by proxy: a family affair, *Child Abuse and Neglect*, 14: 577–86.

Meiselman, K. (1978) *Incest*. San Francisco, CA: Jossey Bass.

Melton, G. and Flood, M. (1994) Research policy and child maltreatment: developing the scientific foundation for effective protection of children, *Child Abuse and Neglect*, 18 (supplement 1): 1–28.

Merrick, D. (1996) *Social Work and Child Abuse*. London: Routledge.

Michenbaum, D. (1977) *Cognitive Behavior Modification: An Integrative Approach*. New York: Plenum Press.

Miller, A. (1985) *Thou Shalt Not Be Aware*. London: Pluto Press.

Minuchin, S. (1974) *Families and Family Therapy*. Cambridge, MA: Harvard University Press.

Mitchell, J. (1974) *Psychoanalysis and Feminism*. London: Allen Lane.

Montagu, A. (1980) *Sociobiology Reexamined*. Oxford: Oxford University Press.

Montgomery, J. (1989) The emotional abuse of children, *Family Law*, 19: 25–9.

Montgomery, S. (1982) Problems in the perinatal prediction of child abuse, *British Journal of Social Work*, 12: 189–96.

Morrison, T., Erooga, M. and Beckett, R. (1994) *Sexual Offending Against Children: Assessment and Treatment of Male Abusers*. London: Routledge.

Morton, N. and Browne, K. (1998) Theory and observation of attachment and its relation to child maltreatment: a review, *Child Abuse and Neglect*, 22: 1093–104.

Mrazek, P. and Mrazek, D. (1987) Resilience in child maltreatment victims: a conceptual exploration, *Child Abuse and Neglect*, 11: 357–66.

Mrazek, P., Lynch, M. and Ben-Tovim, A. (1983) Sexual abuse of children in the UK, *Child Abuse and Neglect*, 7: 147–53.

Mueller, E. and Silverman, N. (1989) Peer relations in maltreated children, in D. Cicchetti and V. Carlson (eds) *Child Maltreatment: Theory and Research on the Causes and Consequences of Child Abuse and Neglect*. Cambridge: Cambridge University Press.

Mullender, A. and Morley, R. (1994) *Children Living with Domestic Violence: Putting Men's Abuse of Women on the Child Care Agenda*. London: Whiting and Birch.

Munro, E. (1999) Protecting children in an anxious society, *Health Risk and Society*, 1: 117–27.

Murphy, J., Jenkins, J., Newcombe, R. and Sibert, J. (1981) Objective birth data and the prediction of child abuse, *Archives of Disease in Childhood*, 56: 295–7.

Murphy, J., Jellinek, M., Quinn, D. *et al.* (1991) Substance abuse and serious child mistreatment: prevalence, risk and outcome in a court sample, *Child Abuse and Neglect*, 15: 197–211.

Murphy-Beaman, V. (1994) A conceptual framework for thinking about risk assessment and case management in child protective services, *Child Abuse and Neglect*, 18: 193–201.

Nash, C. and West, D. (1985) Sexual molestation of young girls, in D. West (ed.) *Sexual Victimisation*. Aldershot: Gower.

National Center on Child Abuse and Neglect (NCCAN) (1981, 1986) *National Study of the Incidence and Severity of Child Abuse and Neglect*. Washington, DC: NCCAN.

National Society for the Prevention of Cruelty to Children (NSPCC) (1996) *Childhood Matters: The Report of the National Commission of Inquiry into the Prevention of Child Abuse. Vol. 1*. London: HMSO.

National Society for the Prevention of Cruelty to Children (1999) *Out of Sight: NSPCC Report on Deaths from Abuse: 1973–1998*. London: NSPCC.

Nelson, B. (1984) *Making an Issue of Child Abuse: Political Agenda Setting for Social Problems*. Chicago: University of Chicago Press.

Nelson, S. (1987) *Incest: Fact and Myth*. Edinburgh: Strathmullion.

Neursten, L., Goldering, J. and Carpenter, S. (1984) Non-sexual transmission of sexually transmitted diseases: an infrequent occurrence, *Pediatrics*, 74: 67–76.

Newberger, C. and White, K. (1989) Cognitive foundations for parental care, in D. Cicchetti and V. Carlson (eds) *Child Maltreatment: Theory and Research on the Causes and Consequences of Child Abuse and Neglect*. Cambridge: Cambridge University Press.

Newlands, M. and Emery, J. (1991) Child abuse and cot deaths, *Child Abuse and Neglect*, 15: 275–8.

Newson, J. and Newson, E. (1989) *The Extent of Parental Physical Punishment in the UK*. London: Approach.

Nobes, G. and Smith, M. (1997) Physical punishment of children in two-parent families, *Clinical Child Psychology and Psychiatry*, 2: 271–81.

Oates, R. (1996) Is it time to have another look at the medical model?, *Child Abuse and Neglect*, 20: 3–5.

Oates, R. and Bross, D. (1995) What have we learned about treating child physical abuse? A literature review of the last decade, *Child Abuse and Neglect*, 19: 463–73.

Oates, R., Peacock, A. and Forrest, D. (1984) The development of abused children, *Developmental Medicine and Child Neurology*, 26: 649–56.

Oates, R., Forrest, D. and Peacock, A. (1985) Self-esteem of abused children, *Child Abuse and Neglect*, 9: 159–63.

O'Hagan, K. (1989) *Working with Child Sexual Abuse*. Milton Keynes: Open University Press.

O'Hagan, K. and Dillenberger, K. (1995) *The Abuse of Women in Childcare Work*. Buckingham: Open University Press.

Oliver, J. (1985) Successive generations of child maltreatment, *British Journal of Psychiatry*, 147: 484–90.

Ong, B. (1985) The paradox of 'wonderful children': the case of child abuse, *Early Child Development and Care*, 21: 91–106.

Orme, T. and Rimmer, J. (1981) Alcoholism and child abuse: a review, *Journal of Studies on Alcohol*, 42: 273–87.

Ostbloom, N. and Crase, S. (1980) A model for conceptualising child abuse causation and intervention, *Social Casework*, 61: 164–72.

Ounsted, C., Roberts, J., Gordon, M. and Milhgan, B. (1982) The fourth goal of perinatal medicine, *British Medical Journal*, 284: 879–82.

Packman, J. (1975) *The Child's Generation: Child Care Policy from Curtis to Houghton*. Oxford: Blackwell.

Packman, J. (1986) *Who Needs Care?* Oxford: Blackwell.

Parker, H. and Parker, S. (1986) Father–daughter sexual abuse: an emerging perspective, *American Journal of Orthopsychiatry*, 56: 531–49.

Parker, H. J., Bakx, K. and Newcombe, R. (1988) *Living with Heroin: The Impact of a Drugs Epidemic on an English Community*. Milton Keynes: Open University Press.

Parton, N. (1979) The natural history of child abuse: a study in social problem definition, *British Journal of Social Work*, 9: 431–51.

Parton, N. (1981) Child abuse, social anxiety and welfare, *British Journal of Social Work*, 11: 391–414.

Parton, N. (1985) *The Politics of Child Abuse*. London: Macmillan.

Parton, N. (1990) Taking child abuse seriously, in The Violence against Children Study Group, *Taking Child Abuse Seriously*. London: Unwin Hyman.

Parton, N. (1991) *Governing the Family: Child Care, Child Protection and the State*. London: Macmillan.

Parton, N. (1996) Child protection, family support and social work: a critical appraisal of the Department of Health Studies in Child Protection, *Child and Family Social Work*, 11: 3–11.

Parton, N. (1997) *Child Protection and Family Support: Tensions, Contradictions and Possibilities*. London: Routledge.

Parton, N., Thorpe, D. and Wattam, C. (1996) *Child Protection, Risk and the Moral Order*. London: Macmillan.

Paterson, C. and McAllion, S. (1989) Osteogenesis imperfecta and the differential diagnosis of child abuse, *British Medical Journal*, 299: 1451–4.

Pavlov, I. (1927) *Conditioned Reflexes: An Investigation of the Physiological Activity of the Cerebral Cortex*. Oxford: Oxford University Press.

Pelton, L. (1978) Child abuse and neglect: the myth of classlessness, *American Journal of Orthopsychiatry*, 48: 608–17.

Peters, J. (1976) Children who are victims of sexual assault and the psychology of offenders, *American Journal of Psychotherapy*, 30: 395–421.

Pfohl, S. (1977) The 'discovery' of child abuse, *Social Problems*, 24: 310–23.

Pierce, R. and Pierce, L. (1985) The sexually abused child: a comparison of male and female victims, *Child Abuse and Neglect*, 9: 191–9.

Pincus, A. and Minahan, A. (1973) *Social Work Practice: Models and Methods*. Itasca, IL: Peacock.

Plumb, J. (1975) The new world of children in eighteenth century England, *Past and Present*, 67: 64–95.

Polansky, N., DeSaix, C. and Sharlin, S. (1972) *Child Neglect: Understanding and Reaching the Parents*. New York: Child Welfare League of America.

Polansky, N., Chalmers, M., Buttenweiser, E. and Williams, D. (1979) The isolation of the neglectful family, *American Journal of Orthopsychiatry*, 49: 149–52.

Polansky, N., Ammons, P. and Weathersby, B. (1983) Is there an American standard of child care?, *Social Work*, 28: 341–6.

Pollock, L. (1983) *Forgotten Children: Parent–Child Relations from 1500 to 1900*. Cambridge: Cambridge University Press.

Porter, R. (ed.) (1984) *Child Sexual Abuse within the Family*. London: Tavistock.

Pringle, K. (1998) *Children and Social Welfare in Europe*. Buckingham: Open University Press.

Pritchard, C. (1992) Children's homicide as an indicator of effective child protection: a comparative study of Western European statistics, *British Journal of Social Work*, 22: 663–84.

Pritchard, C. (1996) Search for an indicator of effective child protection in a reanalysis of child homicide in the major western countries 1973–1992: a response to Lindsey and Trocme and Macdonald, *British Journal of Social Work*, 26: 545–63.

Read, J. (1998) Child abuse and severity of disturbance among adult psychiatric patients, *Child Abuse and Neglect*, 22: 359–68.

Reavley, W. and Gilbert, M. (1979) The analysis and treatment of child abuse by behavioral psychotherapy, *Child Abuse and Neglect*, 3: 509–14.

Reder, P., Duncan, S. and Gray, M. (1993) *Beyond Blame: Child Abuse Tragedies Revisited*. London: Routledge.

Reite, M. (1987) Infant abuse and neglect: lessons from the laboratory, *Child Abuse and Neglect*, 11: 347–55.

Rivara, F. (1985) Physical abuse in children under 2: a study of therapeutic outcomes, *Child Abuse and Neglect*, 9: 81–7.

Roberts, J. (1988) Why are some families more vulnerable to child abuse?, in K. Browne, C. Davies and P. Stratton (eds) *Early Prediction and Prevention of Child Abuse*. Chichester: Wiley.

Roberts, J. and Taylor, C. (1993) Sexually abused children and young people speak out, in L. Waterhouse (ed.) *Child Abuse and Child Abusers: Protection and Prevention*. London: Jessica Kingsley.

Roberts, J., Lynch, M. and Golding, J. (1980) Postneonatal mortality in children from abusing families, *British Medical Journal*, 281: 102–4.

Rorty, M., Yager, J. and Rossotto, E. (1995) Aspects of childhood physical punishment and family environmental correlates in bulimia nervosa, *Child Abuse and Neglect*, 19: 659–67.

Rose, L. (1986) *The Massacre of the Innocents*. London: Routledge and Kegan Paul.

Rose, L. (1991) *The Erosion of Childhood: Child Oppression in Britain 1860–1918*. London: Routledge.

Rowe, J. and Lambert, L. (1973) *Children Who Wait*. London: ABAFA (Association of British Agencies for Fostering and Adoption).

Rush, F. (1980) *The Best Kept Secret*. Englewood Cliffs, NJ: Prentice-Hall.

Russell, D. (1984) *Sexual Exploitation: Rape, Child Sexual Abuse and Workplace Harrassment*. Beverly Hills, CA: Sage.

Russell, D. (1986) *The Secret Trauma: Incest in the Lives of Girls and Women*. New York: Basic Books.

Rutter, M. (1978) *Maternal Deprivation Reassessed*. Harmondsworth: Penguin.

Rutter, M. (1985) Resilience in the face of adversity: protective factors and resistance to psychiatric disorder, *British Journal of Psychiatry*, 147: 598–611.

Sack, W., Mason, R. and Higgins, J. (1985) The single-parent family and abusive child punishment, *American Journal of Orthopsychiatry*, 55: 253–9.

Sahlins, M. (1977) *The Use and Abuse of Biology*. London: Tavistock.

Scarre, G. (1980) Children and paternalism, *Philosophy*, 55: 117–24.

Scott, M. (1989) *A Cognitive-behavioural Approach to Clients' Problems*. London: Tavistock.

Seagull, E. (1987) Social support and child maltreatment: a review of the evidence, *Child Abuse and Neglect*, 11: 41–52.

Seebohm, F. (1968) *Report of the Committee on Local Authority and Allied Personal Social Services*, Cmnd 3703. London: HMSO.

Seed, P. (1973) *The Expansion of Social Work in Britain*. London: Routledge & Kegan Paul.

Shahar, S. (1990) *Childhood in the Middle Ages*. London: Routledge.

Shapiro Gonzalez, L., Waterman, J., Kelly, R., McCord, J. and Oliveri, M. (1993) Children's patterns of disclosure and recantations of sexual and ritualistic abuse allegations in psychotherapy, *Child Abuse and Neglect*, 17: 281–9.

Sharland, E., Seal, H., Croucher, M., Aldgate, J. and Jones, D. (1996) *Professional Intervention in Child Sexual Abuse*. London: HMSO.

Sharpe, J. (1984) *Crime in Early Modern England 1550–1750*. London: Longman.

Shorter, E. (1976) *The Making of the Modern Family*. London: Collins.

Silbert, M. and Pines, A. (1981) Sexual child abuse as an antecedent to prostitution, *Child Abuse and Neglect*, 10: 283–91.

Sinclair, I. and Gibbs, I. (1998) *Children's Homes: A Study in Diversity*. Chichester: Wiley.

Sivan, A., Schor, D., Koeppi, G. and Noble, L. (1988) Interaction of normal children with anatomical dolls, *Child Abuse and Neglect*, 12: 295–304.

Skinner, A. (1992) *Another Kind of Home: A Review of Residential Child Care*. Edinburgh: HMSO.

Skinner, A. and Castle, R. (1969) *78 Battered Children: A Retrospective Study*. London: NSPCC.

Skinner, B. (1953) *Science and Human Behaviour*. Basingstoke: Collier Macmillan.

Sluckin, W., Herbert, M. and Sluckin, A. (1983) *Maternal Bonding*. Oxford: Blackwell.

Smith, J. (1984) Non-accidental injury to children 1: a review of behavioural intervention, *Behaviour Research and Therapy*, 22: 331–47.

Smith, J. and Rachman, S. (1984) Non-accidental injury to children II: a controlled evaluation of a behavioural management programme, *Behaviour Research and Therapy*, 22: 349–66.

Smith, P. (1991) The child's voice, *Children and Society*, 5: 58–66.

Smith, S. (1975) *The Battered Child Syndrome*. London: Butterworth.

Smith, S., Hanson, R. and Noble, S. (1974) Social aspects of the Battered Baby Syndrome, *British Journal of Psychiatry*, 125: 568–82.

Social Services Inspectorate (SSI) (1988) *Report of an Inspection of Melanie Klein House CHE by the Social Services Inspectorate, London. July 1988*. London: Department of Health.

Social Services Inspectorate (1994) *The Child, the Court and the Video: A Study of the Implementation of the Memorandum of Good Practice on Video Interviewing of Child Witnesses*. London: Department of Health.

Social Services Inspectorate, Wales and Social Information Systems (1991) *Accommodating Children: A Review of Children's Homes in Wales*. Cardiff: Welsh Office.

Somerset Area Review Committee (1977) *Report of the Review Panel Appointed by Somerset Area Review Committee to Consider the Case of Wayne Brewer*. Taunton: Somerset Area Review Committee.

Sommerville, J. (1982) *The Rise and Fall of Childhood*. Beverly Hills, CA: Sage.

Southall, D., Plunkett, M., Banks, M., Falkov, A. and Samuels, M. (1997) Covert video recordings of life-threatening child abuse: lessons for child protection, *Pediatrics*, 100: 735–60.

Stafford-Clark, D. (1965) *What Freud Really Said*. London: McDonald.

Staffordshire (County Council) (1991) *The Pindown Experience and the Protection of Children. The Report of the Staffordshire Child Care Inquiry 1990*. Stafford: Staffordshire County Council.

Stanley, N. (1999) The institutional abuse of children: an overview of policy and practice, in N. Stanley, J. Manthorpe and B. Penhale, *Institutional Abuse: Perspectives across the Life Course*. London: Routledge.

Steele, B. (1986) Notes on the lasting effects of early child abuse throughout the life cycle, *Child Abuse and Neglect*, 10: 283–91.

Steele, B. and Pollock, C. (1974) A psychiatric study of parents who abuse infants and small children, in R. Helfer and C. Kempe (eds) *The Battered Child*, 2nd edn. Chicago: University of Chicago Press.

Stevenson, O. (1998) *Neglected Children: Issues and Dilemmas*. Oxford: Blackwell.

Stocks, T. (1988) Has family violence decreased? A reassessment of the Straus and Gelles data, *Journal of Marriage and the Family*, 50: 281–91.

Stone, L. (1977) *The Family, Sex and Marriage in England 1500–1800*. London: Weidenfeld & Nicolson.

Straus, M. (1979) Family patterns and child abuse in a nationally representative sample, *Child Abuse and Neglect*, 3: 213–25.

Straus, M. (1994) *Beating the Devil Out of Them: Corporal Punishment in American Families*. New York: Lexington Books.

Straus, M. and Gelles, R. (1986) Societal change and change in family violence from 1975 to 1985 as revealed by 2 national surveys, *Journal of Marriage and the Family*, 48: 465–79.

Straus, M., Gelles, R. and Steinmetz, K. (1980) *Behind Closed Doors: Violence in the American Family*. New York: Anchor Press.

Stubbs, P. (1989) Developing anti-racist practice – problems and possibilities, in H. Blagg, J. A. Hughes and C. Wattam (eds) *Child Sexual Abuse*. London: Longman.

Sweet, J. and Resick, P. (1979) The maltreatment of children: a review of theories and research, *Journal of Social Issues*, 35: 40–59.

Sydie, R. (1987) *Natural Women, Cultured Men*. Milton Keynes: Open University Press.

Thane, P. (1981) Childhood in history, in M. King (ed.) *Childhood, Welfare and Society*. London: Batsford.

Theringer, D., Burrows Horton, C. and Millea, S. (1990) Sexual abuse and exploitation of children and adults with mental retardation and other handicaps, *Child Abuse and Neglect*, 14: 301–12.

Thoburn, J., Lewis, A. and Shemmings, D. (1995) *Paternalism or Partnership? Family Involvement in the Child Protection Process*. London: HMSO.

Thomas, T. (1996) Covert video surveillance: an assessment of the Staffordshire protocol, *Journal of Medical Ethics*, 22: 22–5.

Thorpe, D. (1994) *Evaluating Child Protection*. Buckingham: Open University Press.

Thyen, U., Thiessen, R. and Heisohn-Krug, M. (1995) Secondary prevention: serving families at risk, *Child Abuse and Neglect*, 19: 1337–47.

Tilly, L., Fuchs, R., Kertzer, D. and Ransel, D. (1992) Child abandonment in European history: a symposium, *Journal of Family History*, 17: 1–22.

Tingus, K., Heger, A., Foy, D. and Leskin, G. (1996) Factors associated with entry into therapy for children evaluated for sexual abuse, *Child Abuse and Neglect*, 20: 63–8.

Tong, L., Oates, K. and McDowell, M. (1987) Personality development following sexual abuse, *Child Abuse and Neglect*, 11: 371–83.

Toro, P. (1982) Developmental effects of child abuse and neglect: a review, *Child Abuse and Neglect*, 6: 423–31.

Treacher, A. and Carpenter, J. (1984) *Using Family Therapy: A Guide for Practitioners in Different Professional Settings*. Oxford: Blackwell.

Truesdell, D., McNeil, J. and Deschner, J. (1986) Incidence of wife abuse in incestuous families, *Social Work*, 31: 138–40.

Tunstill, J. (1997) Implementing the family support clauses of the 1989 Children Act: legislative, professional and organisational obstacles, in N. Parton (ed.) *Child Protection and Family Support: Tensions, Contradictions and Possibilities*. London: Routledge.

Tyler, A. and Brassard, M. (1984) Abuse in the investigation and treatment of intrafamilial child sexual abuse, *Child Abuse and Neglect*, 8: 47–53.

Tymchuk, A. and Andron, L. (1990) Mothers with mental retardation who do or do not abuse their children, *Child Abuse and Neglect*, 14: 313–23.

Utting, Sir W. (1991) *Children in the Public Care: A Review of Residential Child Care*. London: HMSO.

Utting, Sir W. (1997) *People Like Us: The Report of the Review of the Safeguards for Children Living Away from Home*. London: HMSO.

Wald, M. (1982) State intervention on behalf of endangered children: a proposed legal response, *Child Abuse and Neglect*, 6: 3–45.

Wald, M. and Woolverton, M. (1990) Risk assessment: the emperor's new clothes?, *Child Welfare*, 69: 483–511.

Waller, G. (1994) Childhood sexual abuse and borderline personality disorder in eating disorders, *Child Abuse and Neglect*, 18: 97–102.

Wandsworth (London Borough of) (1990) *Report of the Inquiry into the Death of Stephanie Fox*. London: London Borough of Wandsworth.

Wardhaugh, J. and Wilding, P. (1993) Towards an explanation of the corruption of care, *Critical Social Policy*, 37: 4–31.

Warner, N. (1992) *Choosing with Care: The Report of the Committee of Inquiry into the Selection, Development and Management of Staff in Children's Homes*. London: HMSO.

Waterhouse, L. (ed.) (1993) *Child Abuse and Child Abusers: Protection and Prevention*. London: Jessica Kingsley.

Waterhouse, L. and Carnie, J. (1992) Assessing child protection risk, *British Journal of Social Work*, 22: 47–60.

Welch, S. and Fairburn, C. (1996) Childhood sexual and physical abuse as risk factors for the development of bulimia nervosa: a community-based case control study, *Child Abuse and Neglect*, 20: 633–42.

West, D. and Farrington, D. (1977) *The Delinquent Way of Life: Third Report of the Cambridge Study in Delinquent Development*. London: Heinemann.

Westcott, H. (1993) *Abuse of Children and Adults with Disabilities*. London: NSPCC.

White, I. and Hart, K. (1995) *Report of the Management of Child Care in the London Borough of Islington*. London: London Borough of Islington.

White, K., Benedict, M., Wulff, L. and Kelley, M. (1987) Physical disabilities as risk factors for child maltreatment: a selected review, *American Journal of Orthopsychiatry*, 54: 530–43.

Whitmore, E., Kramer, J. and Knutson, J. (1993) The association between punitive childhood experiences and hyperactivity, *Child Abuse and Neglect*, 17: 357–66.

Wiedemann, T. (1989) *Adults and Children in the Roman Empire*. London: Routledge.

Wiehe, V. (1989) Child abuse: an ecological perspective, *Early Child Development and Care*, 42: 141–5.

Wild, N. (1986) Sexual abuse of children in Leeds, *British Medical Journal*, 292: 1113–16.

Wilson, E. (1975) *Sociobiology: The New Synthesis*. Cambridge, MA: Harvard University Press.

Wilson, S. (1984) The myth of motherhood a myth: the historical view of European child rearing, *Social History*, 9: 181–98.

Wohl, A. (1978) Sex and the single room: incest among the Victorian working classes, in A. Wohl (ed.) *The Victorian Family*. London: Croom Helm.

Wolfe, D. (1985) Child-abusive parents: an empirical review and analysis, *Psychological Bulletin*, 97: 462–82.

Wolfe, D., Sandler, J. and Kaufman, K. (1981) A competency-based parent training program for child abusers, *Journal of Consulting and Clinical Psychology*, 49: 633–40.

Wolff, R. (1981) Origins of child abuse and neglect within the family, *Child Abuse and Neglect*, 5: 973–9.

Wolock, L. and Horowitz, B. (1984) Child maltreatment as a social problem: the neglect of neglect, *American Journal of Orthopsychiatry*, 54: 530–43.

Woodroofe, K. (1962) *From Charity to Social Work in England and the United States*. London: Routledge & Kegan Paul.

Wurr, C. and Partridge, I. (1996) The prevalence of a history of childhood sexual abuse in an acute adult inpatient population, *Child Abuse and Neglect*, 20: 867–72.

Yelloly, M. (1980) *Social Work Theory and Psychoanalysis*. New York: Van Nostrand Reinhold.

Young, L. (1964) *Wednesday's Child: A Study of Child Neglect and Abuse*. New York: McGraw-Hill.

Younghusband, E. (1978) *Social Work in Britain 1950–1975*. London: Allen & Unwin.

Zimrin, H. (1986) A profile of survival, *Child Abuse and Neglect*, 10: 339–49.

INDEX